Lillian Carter

ALSO BY GRANT HAYTER-MENZIES
AND FROM MCFARLAND

Mrs. Ziegfeld:
The Public and Private Lives of Billie Burke (2009)

Charlotte Greenwood: The Life and Career of
the Comic Star of Vaudeville, Radio and Film (2007)

Lillian Carter

A Compassionate Life

Grant Hayter-Menzies

Foreword by President Jimmy Carter

McFarland & Company, Inc., Publishers
Jefferson, North Carolina

LIBRARY OF CONGRESS CATALOGUING-IN-PUBLICATION DATA

Hayter-Menzies, Grant, 1964–
    Lillian Carter : a compassionate life / Grant Hayter-Menzies ;
foreword by President Jimmy Carter.
        p.   cm.
    Includes bibliographical references and index.

    ISBN 978-0-7864-9719-5 (softcover : acid free paper) ∞
    ISBN 978-1-4766-1933-0 (ebook)

    1. Carter, Lillian, 1898–1983.   2. Mothers of presidents—
United States—Biography.   3. Carter, Jimmy, 1924—Family.
4. Nurses—United States—Biography.   5. Women civil rights
workers—Georgia—Biography.   6. Plains (Ga.)—Biography.
I. Title.

E874.C375H49 2015
973.926092—dc23
[B]   2014041008

BRITISH LIBRARY CATALOGUING DATA ARE AVAILABLE

On the cover: Lillian Carter on her return visit to India in 1977
(Peace Corps)

Printed in the United States of America

McFarland & Company, Inc., Publishers
  Box 611, Jefferson, North Carolina 28640
    www.mcfarlandpub.com

In memory of my mother
and my grandmother

To Les and Freddie
with love

Table of Contents

Foreword

by President Jimmy Carter

I had planned to spend my life as a career naval officer, but changed my mind when my father died. At his deathbed in 1953, I realized how he had been of benefit to so many people in our small town of Plains and decided to return home and emulate him in every way I could. His was an example that led me into local, state and national politics. My mother's life was changed just as profoundly.

She was a registered nurse, and she had devoted her service to the poorest people among our neighbors, many of them in black families. Unlike others in our segregated Southern community, she never honored the racial or cultural distinctions. My father's death, while devastating to her, freed her to expand her life and to become everything she was meant to be.

As a widow, my mother embarked on a life of purpose which took her far from Plains. A seven-year stint as house mother at Auburn University for a fraternity rumored to be the most hell-raising of any in the state (her reason for choosing it) followed. Her fierce loyalty, ability to share a drink, and her unconditional affection stamped her in the hearts of every member of the fraternity. For Mother, looking after these young men was only the beginning. She then spent three years managing a nursing home for a friend, and in 1964 she became county campaign manager for President Lyndon B. Johnson, running a daily gauntlet of racist slurs scrawled across the sides of her Cadillac. In these fractious years, Mama was in her element.

Sitting up in bed watching television one night in 1966, Mama's attention was grabbed by an advertisement slogan for the Peace Corps that seemed to challenge her to action: "Age is no barrier." At 68, Mother joined the Peace Corps and served as a public health volunteer in Vikhroli, thirty miles outside Mumbai. Assigned to work with untouchables (*dalits*), she dismayed upper caste Indians by doing the kind of work untouchables did. She treated leprosy patients, cleaned up human excrement, and confronted India's own traditional segregation policies by openly eating and socializing with untouchables, at the same time introducing to these marginalized people the concept of equal rights for wives and daughters in and out of the home. She learned the languages and the belief systems of her hosts, reading the *Baghavad Gita* and talking with famous holy men. During those years in India, Mama went from middle-class white Southern woman with a fur coat and diamond rings to barefoot caregiver who, as she had done in Plains decades before, counted no costs in bringing medicines and medical care to people for whom few other people cared.

Mother returned to Atlanta in 1968 with ten cents to her name, so thin we were shocked at the sight of her. But she had changed inside as well as outside. She left part of her heart in India—with the rest of it she determined to dedicate her life to making the world a better place for all people not so fortunate as she.

Her energy and purpose grew with my political aspirations, from my governorship of Georgia in 1971 to my run for the White House in 1976. Mama became one of the Carter campaign's most formidable public relations weapons. As much a fixture in her rocking chair at the Plains campaign headquarters as she was stumping across the nation, rubbing elbows with the leading lights of show business and literature and domineering talk shows with her inimitable style, my mother saw the unimaginable become reality in 1976 when I was elected President of the United States. Through her influence as First Mother, she would see her personal humanitarian values put into global action. Mama not only called on governments to address racism, poverty and health care, but came out for gay rights at a time when few public figures had the courage to do so.

She also turned out to be a magnetic and effective ambassador. I often sent her in my place to far-flung locales to represent the White House; she toured African nations, where rulers rolled out red carpets for the white-haired lady in blue pantsuits, knowing she might find solutions to their problems. Her greatest overseas journey was back to Vikhroli in 1977, where the little gardener's daughter she had taught to read was a top scholar at her university (and one day a university president), and where Mama was celebrated by thousands who greeted her as "Lilly behn"—*our sister Lilly*.

When Rosalynn and I set up The Carter Center in Atlanta as an agency to support and protect human rights and as a neutral setting for conflict resolution, we called on Mother to advise us on medical care needs in third world societies. A crucial part of the Center's mission statement—to be "guided by a fundamental commitment to human rights and the alleviation of human suffering"—could be her life's credo.

By the time she died in 1983, Mama had moved from personality to legend—"First Mother of the World," proclaimed the press. The Carter Center's partner, Emory University, established the Lillian Carter Center for International Nursing in honor of her work in India, while the Peace Corps created the Lillian Carter Award honoring outstanding senior volunteers. Numerous other awards and scholarships have been set up in her name. But above all, the ideals she fostered in her children on a remote farm in southwest Georgia continue to empower and inspire countless individuals through all the people she touched during her long life.

Not only was age no barrier to my mother. Her life was an example of how barriers of color, gender or creed were there to be broken. "Dare to do the things and reach for goals in your own lives that have meaning for you as individuals," Mama wrote in 1968 from India, in a letter addressed to her children but just as applicable to children everywhere, "doing as much as you can for everybody, but not worrying if you don't please everyone."

Mama lived not to please, but to heal.

Preface

I never met Lillian Carter in person. But long before I came to know her family or see the farm where she lived or the community where she nursed during the Great Depression, I was introduced to her through another woman who shared her ideals: my grandmother Nina.

Born on an east Texas farm in 1913, the summer Lillian Gordy turned fifteen, Nina Lewis Strawser had lived between two different eras. "I seem to be sitting astraddle of the fence of time," she wrote in a 1970 essay, "and looking on both sides of it at once, seeing things in retrospect as well as prospect."[1] She had entered life just as the last of the antebellum south was dying out. In her childhood, my grandmother knew very old relatives who remembered family fields worked by slaves. There was for her no romance in looking back at old Dixieland. "Had I been alive then," my grandmother told me of her family's enslaved people, "I would have let them all go."

My grandmother could not bear to see the powerless of society be made to suffer by the powerful, whether blacks oppressed in the south of her girlhood or the dispossessed poor she wrote of in a memoir of her life as a young Depression bride. These experiences fueled her compassion years later for the plight of migrant farm workers in California's Central Valley; she avidly followed the triumphs of their defender Cesar Chavez. For my grandmother, faith in the triumph of good over evil came from her devout religious beliefs. Part, too, came from personal knowledge of how to face adversity and overcome. Leaders like the Rev. Dr. Martin Luther King, Jr., were high on her list, as was a man also honored by Lillian Carter, though he was rarely accorded such respect in the south where both women were born. Like Lillian, my grandmother revered Abraham Lincoln.

A few years before Jimmy Carter was elected president, my grand-mother saved her money to fly out from California to Maryland visit her only son, who had survived the Vietnam War physically if not emotionally. While she was there she spent part of a day in Washington, D.C. My grand-mother loved early American history, in seminal events of which her ances-tors had taken part, and she tried to see as many of the city's historical sites as time allowed. One monument, though, claimed the bulk of her short schedule. For more than an hour, my grandmother sat inside the Lincoln Memorial, meditating on the words engraved on marble like prayers writ large: the Gettysburg Address, the Second Inaugural. Malice toward none. Charity for all. Firmness in the right as God gives us to see the right. A just and lasting peace among ourselves and with all nations. She was inspired by these words not just as the mother of a decorated war veteran but as cit-izen of a nation that had a good deal more healing to do if a just and lasting peace was ever to be achieved.

By the time of the 1976 presidential campaign, my grandmother was not alone in knowing little that was concrete about Democratic candidate Jimmy Carter. But as the campaign progressed, and especially as Miss Lillian made her splash in print and television media, my grandmother felt she could trust the candidate's character through the good works and good humor of his mother. Jimmy Carter's mother had not only joined the Peace Corps as a senior citizen to care for untouchable workers and peasants in the slums of Mumbai, but she had spent her prime years of motherhood nursing black families around Plains, Georgia, at a time when few whites played such a benign role in the lives of black people. Many of the issues both Lillian and Jimmy stood for mattered to my grandmother, too, as they did to women and men across a nation that had suffered the Vietnam War and the Watergate hearings, who remembered the Great Depression and who knew that the time for racial discrimination was over. This majority made Jimmy Carter president in 1976, and my grandmother was proud to be of their number. Though her hopes were sorely tested when Carter lost to Ronald Reagan four years later, she believed in Jimmy more than ever, admiring his and Rosalynn's hands-on philanthropy at home and abroad. Like the Carters, my grandmother believed it was possible to "heal a trou-bled world," as she wrote in an essay inspired by the Vietnam War, "because there can be no peace for a nation until there is peace for the individual, and that peace each must search for and find within himself."[2]

Rosalynn and Jimmy Carter found that peace and that healing which Lillian had first discovered in the dire poverty of rural Georgia and in the suburbs of one of India's richest cities by sharing them with a world desperately needing both—indeed, when they were first preparing the groundwork for The Carter Center (founded in 1982), Lillian's advice was consulted and heeded. The Carter Center's credo of making the world a place where peace has a fighting chance was also Lillian's, as she outlined clearly in a letter sent home from Vikhroli, India, during her service in the Peace Corps. In words which, for me, evoke my grandmother, and say all that needs to be said about The Carter Center's credo, Lillian wrote, "Sharing yourself with others, and accepting their love for you, is the most precious gift of all."[3]

Jimmy Carter's generosity in sharing his mother with me so that I could begin the writing of this book should come as no surprise. Yet I never expected him to agree to my idea; in fact, I gave plenty of leeway for him to refuse me. If you don't want me to touch this, I wrote him, please let me know and I will back off. A few weeks later, his response came. It was to the point but meaningful, just like the man himself. "I welcome you to do it," he told me, and suggested I begin by attending Lillian's induction into the Georgia Women of Achievement hall of fame at Wesleyan College in Macon, Georgia. This was in February 2011, with the induction a month away. I lost no time making last minute flight and hotel arrangements and wrote Jimmy in a note that I planned to be there. When I first met him at a small reception before the induction, the first thing he said, with that smile (and wit) so like his mother's, was "I didn't think you'd really come!"[4] That's a challenge no writer worth his salt could turn down.

The construction of a book like this requires about as many helping hands as are needed for the building of a house. Not just the people who are on site, doing the actual labor, but the many others who contribute to the project from all four corners of the world. All are necessary to helping finish the job that the writer sketched as an architectural elevation which might, just might, actually function as adequate shelter for his subject to live in.

First and foremost I thank Jimmy and Rosalynn Carter, because without them this book could never have been. I first met the Carters at a kitchen table in the house where Lillian and Earl Carter first lived after their marriage, and we had very much a kitchen table conversation, starting with his mother and extending to everything under the sun. Then and during our subsequent visits, I learned a lot about the man Miss Lillian raised. For example, one evening beside a pond outside Plains, as I had a picnic supper with Jimmy and Rosalynn, we talked about women's rights, about which I thought I knew a great deal. "When did women gain the right to vote?" Jimmy suddenly asked me. Proud of a great-grandmother who had been in the forefront of the suffragette movement in San Francisco, I answered that they had done so in 1920. "No, they didn't," he replied, with a smile as rueful as it was "gotcha." "Only white women gained the right to vote in 1920—black women couldn't do so for many years yet. People don't always think about that."[5] He was right; I hadn't thought about it. As his mother might have said, don't ever think there isn't always something more to learn.

Many others have helped me along this journey into the life of Miss Lillian.

I extend special thanks to Kim Carter Fuller, Billy Carter's eldest daughter, who in so many ways is Lillian reincarnate, especially where her loving heart is concerned. (And I thank you, Kim, for that special hour spent at the Pond House.)

From the start, Jill Stuckey has been the kind and generous pilot of my often uncertain ship, bringing me to harbor in so many ways, teaching me what giving is all about. The weekend I spent editing this book under her friendly roof, just across the hall from the Conception Room or out on the porch where the newlywed Lillian and Earl Carter surely sat together of many an evening, gave me valuable insight into their lives and the unique blessings of southern hospitality.

Jan Williams sat me down in the Old Bank Café and shared a wealth of wit and wisdom over sweet iced teas, and she walked me around the old and beautiful workers' cabins near Archery, helping me contemplate and truly appreciate the rich lives of those who had inhabited them.

But for Kenneth H. Thomas, Jr., with whom I started an impromptu conversation about genealogy at Wesleyan College, I might never have gotten my facts straight. Thank you, Ken.

My gratitude goes to Dr. Madhavi Pethe and her brother Milind Vinod, who shared their childhood memories of Lillian in Vikhroli, India, and to Dr. Gyansham Bhatia, who told me what it was like working with the white-haired grandmother and powerhouse nurse from America.

A big thanks to the brothers of Auburn University's Kappa Alpha fraternity—Bill Bassett, Tom Burson, Bill Jordan, Sam Ligon, Tommy Morgan, Jim Rogers—who to a man still revere the woman they know as Miss Lilly, and to Dr. Debbie Shaw of Auburn University for helping me connect with them. And equal gratitude to the Returned Peace Corps Volunteers who frankly and lovingly shared their stories of "Lilly" with me—Dr. Larry Brown, Jules Quinlan, Dr. Gabriel and Ruth Ross, Evangeline Shuler, and Carol Stahl.

My heartfelt appreciation to the staff of the Carter Library at The

Carter Center, especially to the following: Dr. Steven H. Hochman, Mary Ann McSweeney, Pollie Nodine, Brittany Parris, Sara Saunders, Charles Stokeley, Keith Shuler, and James A. Yancey.

Without the generosity of the following, this portrait of Miss Lillian could never have been started let alone completed: David Alsobrook, Anne Yewell Ashton, Steven Borns, Tad Brown, Tina Calhoun, Jack and Elizabeth Carter, Jeff Carter, Sybil Carter, Lynn Chalmers, Ron Counsellor, The Honorable Tom Daschle, Senator for South Dakota, 1987–2005, Lauren Gay, Pheroza Godrej, Rex Granum, Richard Harden, Steven Hunsicker, Rick Hutto, Richard Hyatt, Lenny Jordan, Annette Miller, Mary Minion, Souleymane Ouloguem, Lillian Pickett, Shelli Siebert, John Varner, Johnny Walker (Mr. Wrestling II), Phil Wise, Cindy and Scott Yewell, Ambassador Andrew J. Young, and the people of Plains—from the Jimmy Carter National Historic Site Visitor Center to the businesses along Main Street—who always welcome me like an old friend.

I am grateful to my cousin, Duane Strawser, for sharing his memory of our grandmother's meditation in the Lincoln Memorial, to my cousin Joanne Walker Flowers for her wit and wisdom, and to my siblings, Sean William Menzies and Ronda Menzies, for their support and encouragement. I thank our parents, Glenda and Ronald Menzies, for bringing us up to regard all people as our sisters and brothers and to never fear speaking truth to power. And I am grateful, always and forever, to William Luce.

Special thanks and love to Michele Rubin, who believed in this project from the beginning, and in me long, long before.

PART I. DAUGHTER OF THE SOUTH

Herein lies the tragedy of the age: not that men are poor,—all men know something of poverty; not that men are wicked,—who is good? Not that men are ignorant,—what is Truth? Nay, but that men know so little of men.

—W.E.B. Du Bois, *The Souls of Black Folk*

CHAPTER 1

Bessie Lillian

On September 26, 1978, Lillian Gordy Carter sat in Room 492 in the Old Executive Office Building in Washington, D.C. From the east-facing windows of the mansard-roofed structure that Mark Twain, even in excess-obsessed Gilded Age America, considered the ugliest piece of architecture in the country, you could see the pristine wedding cake of the White House, built in an era when less was more.

Across from Mrs. Carter, whose age-scored visage journalist Orde Coombs described as "somewhere between the cragginess of Lillian Hellman's and the canyons of W.S. Auden's in his last days,"[1] sat bright-eyed 30-something Dr. David Alsobrook. This fellow southerner and member of the Presidential Papers Staff was detailed to interview his subject as part of an oral history project ordered by President Jimmy Carter, Lillian's eldest son. With the recent death of Carter's uncle Alton "Buddy" Carter weighing on him, the president felt time slipping away, and with it the stories that had shaped and colored his increasingly distant childhood.

Alsobrook was lucky to have the president's mother to himself for an hour. Miss Lillian—to use the southern courtesy name by which she was already known across the nation—had turned eighty years old the previous month, and there were few who didn't seek the opportunity to sit a spell with her. Popularity brought problems which were only to multiply as Carter's term progressed. At the little train depot in Plains, Georgia, where Lillian held court during Jimmy Carter's presidential campaign, she had been so in demand that signs had to be nailed up asking enthusiastic visitors to speak to, but not touch, the diminutive white-haired lady smiling from her rocking chair: she had found herself bruised from all the attention.

(Though as Richard Harden, Lillian's frequent aide on her travels, points out, "she never did like to be hugged or kissed, unless it was someone young and attractive.")[2] After Carter's inauguration, his mother was sought after to a degree more appropriate to a rock star than a genteel grandmother from south Georgia. To meet with her required security protocol and careful planning, aside from finding an empty slot in her overcrowded calendar. Lillian had become, in the worn but accurate phrase, a legend in her own time.

Alsobrook had studied at Auburn University, the Alabama institution where Lillian served as colorful and beloved housemother to Kappa Alpha Fraternity from 1956 to 1962. Combined with his Alabama heritage, this gave him an edge as an otherwise unknown interviewer, but Alsobrook found that even an Auburn boy could overstep the line. "I asked her about her childhood growing up in the impoverished South," he remembered, "and when she told me about it I said, 'I know just what you mean, Miss Lillian'—she was so much like my grandmother, I felt I could understand her from that angle. But she looked at me and said, 'No, you *don't* know.' And it's true—what did I know about being a little girl growing up in the South of her childhood?" She'd grown up in a world where women weren't given anything for free, Alsobrook recalled. "She'd seen women in her family struggling to make something of themselves in what was very much a man's world. That was something no *man* could understand."[3]

Keeping this in mind, Alsobrook coaxed her through a series of questions dealing with every facet of her fourscore decades of life—childhood, parents, siblings, education, marriage, motherhood, her work as a nurse, allowing her to answer as she pleased. It was motherhood, of course, which drew greatest interest. What special thing did a mother from Plains, a village set in the peanut and cotton fields of southwest Georgia, do to shape a future President of the United States? The same question had been directed at several presidential mothers, and the answers they gave usually boiled down to three basic ingredients: discipline, compassion, and courage. Famous for the wisecrack, "Sometimes, when I look at my children, I say to myself, 'Lillian, you should have remained a virgin.'" Lillian was not about to make the sort of edifying comment you might have heard from Sara Delano Roosevelt or Ida Truman. "She was never subtle about what she felt," Alsobrook laughs.[4] And she was already highly skilled at playing mind games with reporters, to the extent their probing appeared to deserve it. She had plenty of reason to be wary. Her family had become the subject of increasingly distorted caricatures in the press since Jimmy Carter had taken office—editorial cartoons of hillbillies, straw protruding from ears

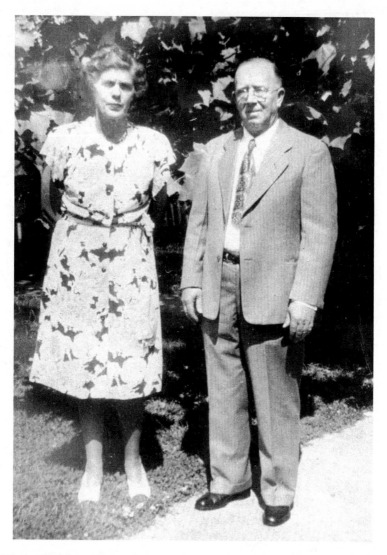

**Lillian and Earl Carter, circa late 1940s. "I have never ceased being lonely for him,"
said Lillian on Earl's death in 1953, "but I've never been lonely for anyone else"
(courtesy Jimmy Carter Presidential Library).**

as they slouched around outhouses and chicken coops—in one of the most
egregious cases of stereotyping ever inflicted on a presidential family. Lillian
was happy to downplay her own middle-class background if it would attract
working-class votes for her son, but when the press went too far she spoke
up, often in riddles that amused or frustrated—or refused to speak to them
at all. It didn't take long for even the greenest journalist to see that this
soft-spoken lady was all too comfortable with being in charge. "Miss Lillian

is afraid of no man," a 98 year old black woman once told a reporter passing through Plains. "She says what's bothering her and, shoot, if you don't like it, she ain't about to ask you why."[5]

It would have been the most natural thing in the world to expect such a woman to take credit for her son's phenomenal political success—her participation in the campaign had certainly helped secure it—and she did state on occasion that meeting her was the next best thing to meeting the president. But Lillian Carter wasn't to be pigeonholed so neatly. It was the children's father, James Earl Carter, Sr., who "taught them there are other places besides Plains...," she insisted. "'Don't stop, study as hard as you can,'" she quoted her husband. "'Hitch your wagon to a star.'"[6] In fact, Lillian spent the better part of the interview talking about Earl, whose tragically early death in 1953 had nearly broken her spirit. She seemed to enjoy relating the information that "he was the kind of Christian who didn't mind if you had a drink," that he danced better "when he was a little high," or that he smiled "just like Jimmy does.... He smiled all day long." She candidly told of their first meeting. "I just didn't like his looks," she confessed, until a family friend, Dr. Sam Wise, insisted she give Earl a chance. She found herself married to a dynamo who did become Plains' leading businessman. "He planned for the future every day of his life," she told Alsobrook, and not just for the future of his own family. He was also, she was careful to say, a constant if unheralded source of support for the disadvantaged of the town—white *and* black.[7]

Only well into the interview, after Alsobrook had slightly increased the pressure, did Lillian comment on her own work for the poor of Plains, most famously among the black sharecroppers who lived around the Carter farm in the rural community of Archery. "I still have letters," she said. "'You were so wonderful to blacks as well as whites,'" went one of them. "'You nursed the blacks.'"[8] Yet she consistently downplayed any notion that she had done anything great, even as a Peace Corps volunteer in India. Strictly speaking, Lillian was no Mother Teresa; her hands-on humanitarian efforts had never extended further than the outskirts of a village, whether the poverty-stricken hovels of Vikhroli outside Mumbai or the poverty-stricken cabins of the black workers on her husband's lands. But as it had taken a village in the deep south to open her eyes and heart to the miseries of institutionalized racism, the plight of Untouchables, India's second-class citizens, and of the non-people India made of its women, moving her to appeal to the wider world in speeches and actions for solutions and, above all, for compassion, a word she spoke like a prayer. Since childhood, Lillian pointed out, "I have been for the underdog. All of my life I've loved to do things for people who couldn't help themselves." When Alsobrook asked her if she had really galloped on horseback to the aid of the little black girl dying of colitis, she vigorously denied it—she'd taken Jimmy's pony cart. She would not permit herself to exaggerate her actions into heroism, and it troubled her when anyone else tried. "I saw people who had nothing," she explained simply, "and I had to help."[9]

It was then, toward the end of Alsobrook's interview, that Lillian did make a statement which, in its unadorned style, spoke directly to just how crucial her personal belief system was to the formation of Jimmy Carter— the Georgia governor who raised both ire and hope in his 1971 inaugural speech by declaring "the time for racial discrimination is over," the former president who, almost forty years later, stated unequivocally that "the practice of religion is the basic cause, or foundation, for other abuses" of the rights of women, who fought to eradicate African diseases unknown in a First World which ignored their existence in the Third.[10]

"I always say people outside Plains love me more than the people in Plains," Lillian explained to Alsobrook. "The blacks love me more than the whites. The Jews love me more than the gentiles. And the Indians love me better than anybody. That's because I have never noticed a color line." Should there ever be a race riot in Plains, she added, "I wouldn't be afraid at all of the blacks, but I might be a little bit afraid of some of the whites." In perhaps the most candid admission she had ever shared with an interviewer, she said simply and starkly, "In my town, I have stood alone."[11]

Jimmy Carter learned from his father the businessman's prudence of working with others to find common solutions, even to reaching out to perceived enemies to start dialogue of benefit to all. From his mother, he learned the difficult art of standing up for what he believed in, regardless of what the majority might think or legislate or of threats of bodily harm— and especially, regardless of the perils embodied in the civil disobedience of standing alone.

"I was Papa's favorite," Lillian insisted. "Everybody will tell you that."[12]

Like his daughter, James Jackson Gordy was a southerner far ahead of his time and place. His liberal beliefs on race and social class, which Lillian absorbed "as if by osmosis",[13] made Gordy a rarity not only in the late nineteenth century, when the "War Between the States" still pained southerners all too keenly, but as a mature man well into the twentieth, when the poisoned fruit of unresolved racism continued to sprout a bumper crop of hatred.

If her father was her social conscience, Lillian's mother, Mary Ida Nicholson Gordy, was her mentor in the gentler realm of compassion. Ida was also an example of the sort of mother Lillian would herself become: fiercely loyal and protective toward her brood, toward each of whom she refused to give more than a strictly equal portion of her love and encouragement.

The Gordys had originally come down from Maryland's eastern shore, where their earliest confirmed forebear, Adrian Gordy, died in 1715. Gordy left the last will and testament of a moderately prosperous man, but as a person he remains undefined as a shadow—one of those ironies of the universe, since obscure as he was, Gordy's gene pool built wiser than he knew. He was the common grandsire not only of President Jimmy Carter but of President Barack Obama—a genealogical legacy appropriate for Lillian Carter. (Another one, just as apropos: Lillian also brought the Carters cousinships to the king of rock 'n' roll, Elvis Presley, and to the founder of Motown, Berry Gordy.)[14]

By the time Lillian's grandfather, James Thomas Gordy, was born in Baldwin County, Georgia in 1828, the family had long been farming the rich red Georgian soil, from which cotton and everything seemed to grow twice as fast as anywhere else. Wilson Gordy, James' father, was to eventually settle at Cusseta in Chattahoochee County, near the Alabama border.[15]

James Thomas was a prosperous farmer and slave-holder near Cusseta when war was declared on April 12, 1861, between the newly minted Confederacy and the Union. He was already the father of three children by his wife Harriet Emily Helms; Lillian's father James Jackson, who was known to family, friends and the census taker as Jim Jack, didn't come along until partway through the Civil War, in 1863, and five more children (all boys) would be born after the conflict. James Thomas's father, Wilson, was more sturdy yeoman than leisured cavalier. Like him, most southern planters did not live in Hollywood's version of the O'Haras' "Tara." Fathers and sons helped field slaves bring in the harvest; mothers and daughters worked alongside slaves in the household. Their plantation houses didn't boast white columns but they were as likely to contain books, a piano or fiddle, ancestral chairs or a table carried carefully over rough frontier trails from some milder place of origin, along with the other niceties made affordable by free slave labor. "Slaveholders understood their rule to be the incarnation of the well-ordered society," wrote Ira Berlin, "which mirrored the well-ordered family." This was the apparently placid life, with its static, safely narrow values and its unequal but no less binding interlocking of family members white and black, that the Gordys knew before war came to alter the landscape of both farm and its people. As much to defend these relationships and the way of life they supported, the Gordys sacrificed to the Confederate cause with their blood: several of Wilson's sons fought in the war and two, Gilbert and William, died in it. James Thomas served the Confederacy as wagon master, having enlisted as a private in Company B, 6th Georgia State Militia, in 1864, the last year of the war. That May, Union General William Tecumseh Sherman began his march from Chattanooga, Tennessee, cutting through the state from Atlanta to Savannah at the coast. If the Gordys were not in the direct line of Sherman's forces or the marauding brigades of "bummers" who burned stored cotton and slaughtered livestock, they were well within hearsay of the horrors of the Confederate prison at Andersonville, where living skeletons that had been Union soldiers lived out their last within the overcrowded stockade. Having lost sons to the "cause"—James Thomas himself had had a lucky escape when his entire company was captured—the Gordys might well have wondered which side could possibly win in such an even contest of inhumanity.[16]

The first sign that the Gordys had left agriculture behind came when James Thomas began supplementing his farming income by serving as county tax collector—the ravaged post-war agrarian economy of the south was still one where government employment could guarantee a wage. Most of the rest of the Georgia Gordys threw in their lot with the professions. Jim Jack's elder brother, Dr. Francis Marion Gordy, became a physician, while a younger brother, Dr. Arthur Gordy, was a dentist and the father of State Senator A. Perry Gordy of Columbus. When interviewed in later life, Lillian and her sisters claimed they had barely known these prominent relatives, and given the distances between Richland and the cities where these men lived, it's understandable that the girls would not have seen them very often. But for reasons probably as much political as anything else, this was a part of her family history that Lillian, during her son's run for president, would sometimes do as much to obfuscate as she would the unwelcome fact of her ancestors' ownership of slaves.[17]

In 1888, Jim Jack married Mary Ida Nicholson in Chattahoochee County. Ida was a mild, hard-working and strongly fibered woman who may have brought the Gordys some abolitionist blood through her mother, Elizabeth Dawson. Elizabeth, who lived in the Gordy house during Lillian's girlhood, was a descendant of Gibson Dawson, appointed in 1837 by a prominent planter of Talbot County, Georgia, to serve as his attorney to safeguard several slaves to Indiana. Once he had brought them there, Dawson sold them, which by Georgia law automatically granted them their freedom. It is not likely a committed supporter of slavery would have involved himself in such an enterprise had he not shared his employer's opinion.[18]

Lillian's younger sister remembered their mother Ida in terms of unalloyed sweetness. "She was a little woman," said Elizabeth Gordy Braunstein. "She had long, brown, straight hair which she fixed in a bun at the back of her neck." And she was, she added, "really the Christian in the family," a characterization with which Lillian concurred. Her mother, she said, "was the type of person who, when the neighbor was sick, she did everything for them."[19] Nor did she ever complain, remembered their youngest sister, Emily Gordy Dolvin, known as Sissy to family and friends. "She could be sick, she could be in the bed, she could be feeling bad, but she was always okay."[20] Though Lillian's future sister-in-law Fanny Gordy would describe compassion as a Gordy trait—"All the Gordys are that way ... they're always doing something for somebody"—it was at least as much a Nicholson trait, too.[21]

Ida needed plenty of Christian fortitude. By the time Bessie Lillian Gordy was born on August 15, 1898, in Richland, a sleepy west Georgia town of square-jawed brick storefronts and placid white-porched cottages located some twenty miles from Cusseta, the Gordys already had six children: Susie, James Albert, Walter Lemuel, James Jackson, Jr., Tom Watson and Annie Lee. On a slender schoolmaster's salary, Jim Jack and Ida had had to make do in a household whose dinner table routinely seated thirteen, not counting guests. The extended family included Ida's mother as well as two orphaned sons of Jim Jack's brother, David Crockett Gordy. In 1902, this seemingly untroubled husband and father had risen from the dinner table and, while the family watched, walked into a nearby room, shut the door, began a suicide note that he didn't finish, and put a bullet through his head.[22] His wife, Sallie Estelle Nicholson, a sister to Ida, had died years before, so the boys—Ralph and Rex—were brought to Jim Jack's home in Richland. For the rest of the time the boys lived with their uncle and aunt, they were protected and nurtured in some respects more than Jim Jack and Ida's own children. Because the boys were Catholics, Lillian remembered how she and her siblings watched with amazement and some derision as their cousins said their prayers in a very different fashion from the way they said their own. But neither Ralph nor Rex had the household's Protestant beliefs pushed on them. Lillian would not always attend church throughout her life. To her, as to her parents, Christianity was an intensely individual affair, not proper for wide discussion (she was not always happy when son Jimmy later highlighted the topic as candidate and president). "I think there's a difference between religion and Christianity," she would announce in later years, to the delight of the press and the disapproval of small minds.[23]

Having given up teaching for the postmaster's job he was to hold for the next several decades in several different places, Jim Jack put Ralph and Rex to work at the post office, teaching them such skills as how to use the telegraph machine. Rex helped deliver RFD mail, the existence of which was entirely due to Jim Jack's political lobbying. Prior to Jim Jack's effort to put it in place, there was no free rural delivery in Georgia. (RFD was generally adopted in the U.S. by 1902.) "When Tom Watson was senator," Emily Dolvin remembered. "Daddy wrote the bill and Tom Watson put it through the Senate," she claimed; Jimmy Carter notes that this is not accurate.[24] Among Elizabeth Braunstein's earliest memories, when she was five or six years old, was that of Rex serving as one of the first rural mail deliverymen. And she remembered him for another, sweeter reason. "I was his favorite," she explained, "so I can remember he bought me some red wool, and had me a little cape thing made of it."[25] Whatever trauma these boys had suffered, living in Ida Gordy's house was healing it.

And home was very much Ida's realm—"She ruled our house," affirmed Lillian.[26] Because Jim Jack was frequently away working, almost everything fell on Ida's shoulders; this was to have a profound influence on her daughters, who were encouraged to take up professions allowing them to be independent of anyone, including men.[27] Lillian and her sisters were in agreement that if Ida had more than enough love to go around, she also had more than a little fire in her, emerging when circumstances warranted. Lillian recalled the time her mother was alerted by daughter Annie Lee, who had run home from school, to tell her that the schoolmaster in Richland was whipping Ralph. This could not have been very long after he and his brother had been orphaned, and it doesn't require a psychologist to figure out why Ralph was getting in trouble at school. Like Lillian's, Ida's was a compassion that had in it a righteous rage. Looking out the schoolhouse window, Lillian watched her furious mother struggle up the road in her "Mother Hubbard" dress, the calico folds flowing around her in the dust. Lillian always remembered how Ida strode into the schoolhouse and stopped the teacher in mid-thrash. "If you hit him another lick," she told him, "I'll give it to you." "She wasn't afraid of anything," Lillian recalled proudly. That included Jim Jack. When Lillian's sister Elizabeth followed her into nursing training, despite Jim Jack's continued opposition Ida secretly helped sew her daughter's uniform and supported her in all her efforts. But maintaining her composure as wife of so mercurial a man had its downside. As Ida told Lillian when her daughter announced her engage-

ment to Earl Carter, the best way to let off steam was to find a field farthest
from the house and scream "Damn" in as loud a voice as she could muster.
She advised Lillian to do the same if life with Earl proved anything like life
with Jim Jack.[28]

If prejudice and judgment were the result of insufficient exposure to
education and, especially, to the rich variety of peoples and faiths of the
world outside Richland, Lillian's open mindedness even as a girl can be
said to have started in her parents' book-filled house. All the family read
(Emily Dolvin claimed to have read seven books in one weekend, likely a
record even for the Gordys), even at the dinner table—not a habit that
would have promoted family togetherness, but one which fostered the vigorous discussions beloved by the family. When they weren't reading over
the dinner dishes, the Gordys used the dining table as a prandial battlefield
of ideas and opinions, debate being an inheritance that seemed to come to
Gordys along with blue eyes.

Jim Jack loved music as much as books, and provided a piano and lessons for his daughters, which they were instructed to take with utter seriousness. Jim Jack wasn't easy to please—long after he had ceased to be a
schoolmaster, a pedagogue's air of authority would never quite leave him.
As Lillian described it, her father "overlooked" her and her siblings' reading
material, making sure it was only of the edifying type. His "overlooking"
was so vigilant that Lillian would venture reading of unapproved materials
while sitting at the piano, where she thought he might not suspect what
she was doing. Jim Jack once almost caught her absorbed by the jailhouse
melodrama *Convict 999*, a novel for which she had paid a whopping ten
cents. As her father approached to ask her why she wasn't practicing, Lillian
was able to hide the novel inside the piano and pick up a copy of the Bible
that always sat atop the instrument. "He said, 'You've read the Bible long
enough,'" Lillian remembered. "'You have to practice.'" So back she went
to her scales, "three hours a day," she recalled.[29]

Lillian favored the jaunty "Twelfth Street Rag" (by composer Euday
L. Brown, once a Kansas City bordello pianist)[30] over the more ladylike
parlor pieces of the period, apparently with Jim Jack's leave. But her sister
Elizabeth was held to a different standard. For tossing off a popular tune
called "My Mama Has Fleas" in her father's presence, she received on her
head an especially resounding example of Jim Jack's habitual punishment
when his children fell out of line: "the blamedest thump," recalled Elizabeth, "you ever saw."[31]

One of the few extant childhood photos of Lillian, taken when she was around eleven or twelve, shows a young lady with smoothly parted dark hair, wearing white eyelet and an expression of intense inquiry that seems to push itself from the Victorian into the modern age, relentlessly questioning. It's easy to see why this girl was the only one of Jim Jack's children to withstand the scrutiny and the pressure of his company. "I didn't always accept what he said as the gospel truth," she told her eldest son, "and would argue with some of his opinions"—something Jim Jack's political cronies in Atlanta probably only ventured to do at their peril. But she knew when to draw back—accurately judging crisis in situations or in people would remain one of her great gifts as nurse and political activist. One of the safer kinds of discussions that she could always have with her father was that dealing with books. "I tried to learn about things that interested him," she recalled. "Sometimes he would give me a book he had just read, and we both looked forward to a fierce discussion about the subject," a reflection of Jim Jack's need to have someone to bounce ideas off of, opportunity for which he probably didn't get enough of in Richland. All taken, he was a father easy for a girl to love, handsome and tall, with penetrating blue eyes, a penchant for bow-ties and for keeping crisply accurate records and notes. It was probably because Lillian had always stood her ground with Jim Jack in any debate, never cowering, that he seems to have held her in as much respect as she held him in awe.[32]

Lillian never knew Jim Jack the schoolmaster. By the time she was old enough to be aware of what her father did for a living, Jim Jack was serving as postmaster of Richland. His was an appointment based not on the merit system we know today but on the political patronage without which nothing got done in those less accountable times. That Jim Jack understood the tricky process of keeping his feet in whatever political storms blew up unawares showed him a master of tacking his sails to the political wind: he held on to his job through whatever party was in power. When Republican Warren Harding was elected President in 1920, lifelong Democrat Jim Jack calmly put in his name for the postmaster position in a nearby town that was, in Jimmy Carter's words, "the only rural Republican stronghold" in the area. Because the job was already taken, Jim Jack was put on a list and given a temporary place as chief revenue agent for the area. He also served as a U.S. marshal for a time, a large part of which involved the destruction of illegal moonshine stills in the area. This was a task many said Jim Jack was eminently qualified for, since he already knew and had sampled the wares of most of them.[33] As Emily Dolvin remembered, it was around this time that Jim Jack learned to drive, though he did so in a most unorthodox manner.[34]

"He never learned to back an automobile," Emily said. As a teenager, she would often drive her father to look for stills to destroy, as his inability to back out of rural roads would have proved a handicap. She remembered that when her father had to drive as far as Albany, fifty odd miles south of Richland, "he had a little black boy who used to meet him at the city limits ... and drive him in." Most of the time, Jim Jack probably took the train to the capital, Atlanta, where he spent a great deal of his time "politicking," as his daughters described it. Whatever his clumsiness behind the wheel of a car, Jim Jack's was the kind of politicking that took not just courage but agility, rather like the moves of Lillian's future favorite boxer, Muhammad Ali. And like Lillian, he never made a safe political choice in his life.[35]

In a part of the south where a man either voted Democrat or didn't vote at all, Jim Jack was drawn to a party that would be fraught with controversy from start to finish, the Populist platform. Born in 1891 out of the fears of rural citizens, mostly farmers, who believed northern Republican business interests were robbing them of a way of life that was all they knew, the Populist Party aimed to get rid of national banking systems, ensure an eight hour work day (an issue that had first flared a century earlier, and would not be implemented by unions and legislation for another twenty five years), reform the civil service, and make several other radical changes to the status quo. The Party even flirted with equal rights for (white) women, who though they would not receive the right to vote until 1920 were welcomed into the Party. It was Jim Jack's friend and near contemporary, Populist Thomas E. Watson, who courted not just poor whites but even more radically, blacks. The latter appeared to be an integrationist stance in the name of unifying the Populist vote and ensuring trustworthy results at the ballot boxes. Whether Watson really wanted blacks to consider themselves equal in this or any other context is debatable. He viewed his boyhood on a plantation surrounded by genial slaves as a kind of golden age destroyed by the Civil War. Like Jim Jack a former schoolmaster, Watson became a lawyer and was to have a tumultuous career in politics, to finally be repudiated by his own party and grow increasingly paranoid about enemies he was sure were out to ruin him. He had reason to question the corruption endemic especially in the black vote, which was highly coerced and tainted by intimidation. But this later led him to adopt a racist attitude that would encompass an imagined Jewish lobby in the north, and linked him by association with the case of the Texas-born Jewish businessman Leo

Frank, who was questionably convicted of raping and murdering a gentile girl in 1914, abducted from the State Penitentiary in Millidgeville and lynched before a cheering crowd in 1915.[36]

Lillian made no bones about her father's attitude to the Watson of later years. "I remember when Tom Watson became such a radical about blacks," recalled Lillian, "the friendship was not strong then."[37] Still, Jim Jack served as Watson's District Three campaign manager, supported him in his political career, and remained connected after Watson had become the sort of man who could call for a reconstitution of the Ku Klux Klan, going to Washington at Watson's invitation, where he and son Tom were entertained to breakfast at the White House. Theirs was the kind of relationship that sometimes occurs between people of diametrically opposite beliefs—as a political junkie, Jim Jack could simply have been fascinated by how in one man the liberal position of Populism could live cheek by jowl with far more conservative views toward blacks, Jews and Catholics. (One writer has even suggested, not entirely tongue in cheek, that Jim Jack was a closet Republican, possibly more dangerous in southwest Georgia then than being a friend of black people.) Perhaps having survived the ruptures of the Civil War and its aftermath, but coming to a different conclusion about it than Watson, Jim Jack was less inclined to hole up in the silo of his beliefs, but rather to test them—not the mark of a person unsure of his convictions. (That said, his grandson Jimmy Carter remembered that Jim Jack resented "the Northern oppressors," who had been a power in the south until 1876.) Where many who fought for civil rights might never deign to sit at the same table as Tom Watson, Jim Jack may have felt that to do so was exactly what was needed to help solve the problem at hand, a method of negotiation for which his presidential grandson would be both lauded and condemned.[38]

Watson seems to have been well aware of the points at which he and Jim Jack were far apart and made an effort to avoid offending him any more than was necessary. In a letter Watson wrote to Jim Jack in January 1916, Watson assures him "that I will not take any stand in the Congressional fight in your district, which will injure or embarrass you in any way."[39] Could this be a reference to Jim Jack's friendships in the black community? "Watson was always a political reformer and a liberal," states Tad Brown of the Watson-Brown Foundation of Thomson, Georgia, which provides educational opportunities to underprivileged youth. These two attributes at the very least would have attracted Jim Jack. "Perhaps that solidified the appeal," Brown says. "Watson was an intellectual. Perhaps Gordy was, too."[40] Jim Jack was also a supreme realist. Alienating the political powers in Atlanta or in Washington could not only have spelled trouble for Jim Jack's job. It could have further marginalized the black friends for whom he served as go-between with the whites who controlled government at the local and national level, whom blacks were forbidden to approach.

Until she left home in 1920, Lillian would spend three years working alongside her father at the post office in Richland. (She later became assistant postmaster.) Thanks to this proximity, she was able to meet some of Jim Jack's more famous friends as well as witness his influence-networking first hand. For instance, Tom Watson dropped by one Sunday when she was helping her father put up the mail. She remembered answering the door to find "a funny looking little man" whose surprise appearance her father greeted "as if Jesus had come for a visit."[41] Ironically, the next day there might be a visit from black friends like African Methodist Episcopal Bishop William Decker Johnson, or later on another of her father's controversial acquaintances, Benjamin J. Davis. Davis was born in Dawson, Georgia to an educated family (his father was editor and publisher of the Atlanta *Independent*), was a student activist at Morehouse College in Atlanta, later became a communist and freedom fighter against racism and was imprisoned during the McCarthy years. It was through a man like Davis, claimed Lillian, and exposure to him and her father's diverse crowd of friends and cronies "that I first began to see blacks as people...."[42]

As Jim Jack Gordy's daughter, it's unlikely Lillian ever saw them as anything else—after all, she was the only member of her family who openly defended Abraham Lincoln, and would be one of the few white people in Plains to do so.[43] Yet it cannot be overemphasized how dangerous it was for anyone, white or black, to cross the color line or to abrogate the status quo so publicly.

In the south of Jim Crow lived a set of laws both unwritten and codified in which the lives of people black and white occupied two separate planes of existence. It was a violation of these laws for a white person to consort socially with black, nearly as strict as the rules fencing off blacks from whites and with some of the same severe penalties for disobeying. People who still criticize the Carter family—singling out Jimmy Carter in particular early in his political career—for not speaking and acting more forcefully and publicly against discrimination in and around Plains are not always taking into account the risks such opposition could entail. As in so many things, Jim Jack was obviously willing to run the risk, which of course was not just to his own neck—the families of whites who showed sympathy toward blacks were just as liable to being harassed—when he invited black friends to dine with him in the rooms behind the post office. But he was discreet. He had to be. He brought the meals in himself from the local hotel restaurant where his guests would not have been allowed to enter, let alone order. And he unstintingly if, again, discreetly, used his political influence help his black friends. Bishop Johnson was one of these.

Johnson was an educated, polished man who had broadened his views through travel and study. He would found the Johnson Home Industrial College in Archery, the black community near the train stop just down the road from the Carter farmhouse, for youth living in the area. These Archery youngsters were lucky. Blacks were excluded from white schools and most opportunities for even a rudimentary education, and Georgia was one of the worst states for funding such schools as existed.[44] Bishop Johnson's son Alvan was even luckier. He attended Harvard University, and on his vacations home always came to talk to Lillian, who delighted in hearing of his experiences at an Ivy League university, especially in her son Jimmy's presence. She wanted Jimmy to profit from this brush with the wonderful world outside Plains, Georgia, she said later.

In the days before his appointment, Johnson was often a visitor to the Gordys' home. He never came in the front door or the back but settled on the neutral territory of the front yard and front porch—neighbors were watching, after all, and it would have done Jim Jack no more good than Johnson to be seen welcoming him into the parlor. They mostly kept in touch with letters. "Papa'd write to him," Lillian remembered, "and he'd get a letter nearly every day about something. [Jim Jack] was helping him to do different things." Johnson wanted to be bishop very much, Lillian affirmed. "I think Papa helped him every way he could in his religious politics," she explained in an interview, adding with her characteristic teasing candor, "Did you know politics had religion?"[45] But even as a bishop, Johnson couldn't break the hidebound rules of Jim Crow. When he wanted to visit Jim Jack, Johnson would make an appointment with him, then direct the driver of his gleaming limousine to park in the front yard of the Gordy home. Jim Jack would come outside when the chauffeur tooted the horn, and both men would have their meeting, the laws not broken but certainly circumvented. On occasion they would even sit together on the front porch, singing hymns. "The King of love my shepherd is," the men sang, "I nothing lack if I am His and He is mine forever."[46] Few racists of Richland would be congratulated for complaining about something so innocent, not to mention devout, as this. And Jim Jack's Carter descendants would have enough battles along those lines to fight in the future, not on a front porch but inside, and outside of, the walls of a church.

CHAPTER 2

The Plains of Dura

During the Civil War, many southern towns and cities had converted churches, factories and private homes into makeshift hospitals for the wounded who poured in from the battlefields. The only females considered proper and experienced enough to do work that might expose them to male nakedness and the coarse language brought on by pain were married ladies. These women not only cleaned up blood and vomit, assisted in crude surgeries and read to and wrote letters for the illiterate or the incapacitated, but served to remind the wounded men of the wives, daughters, sisters or mothers they had left often far behind.

Nursing of this kind was considered noble and self-sacrificing, following in the revered footsteps of Florence Nightingale. But fifty years later, when Lillian Gordy told her father she wanted to train to be a nurse, she might as well have asked permission to serve beer in a pub. When Lillian was in her teens, in the second decade of the twentieth century, "nurses were not looked on as being too hot," she recalled when asked about her interest in nursing. "They were kind of looked down upon."[1] This was partly due to the suffragette movement's then-shocking demand for jobs and autonomy for women. In a world where women demanding equality were arrested, jailed, and force-fed during hunger strikes, a woman seeking to join a profession, medicine—long the preserve of males—was suspect. That that profession, on the one hand, allowed her to work with little supervision by men, and exposed her to male patients, and on the other, allowed her to work too closely with doctors who were presumed to take sexual advantage of women like herself, meant that Lillian was asking too much even of her liberal father.

In August 1914, just as Lillian turned sixteen, war broke over the continent of Europe. While the crowned grandchildren of Queen Victoria fired their guns at each other, the United States tried to remain above the fray. President Woodrow Wilson wasn't interested in involving the nation in what was believed to be a European problem. When a German submarine sank the *Lusitania* in 1915 and still others began menacing transatlantic shipping, Wilson's plan to position the United States as a mediator in the conflict drew the country into it. He declared war on Germany on April 2, 1917, and troops were sent overseas. Lillian's interest in becoming a nurse antedated the outbreak of the war, but now that nurses were needed more than ever, she redoubled her efforts on breaking down Jim Jack's opposition. College never interested her, a fact that set her apart from the rest of her family. Of her siblings, only she and a brother managed to avoid university. "I was well-read and I had a good high-school education," she said. "I wanted to get a degree in nursing, but I didn't want to go to college. I hated it." "Something that's within me," Lillian explained, "is helping people who couldn't help themselves." What she really wanted to do was study medicine and become a doctor, a course which, if nursing was already risqué, would have put Lillian beyond the pale of respectability. "I should have been a doctor" was a refrain she would repeat well into old age.[2] She was not wishing for something that had never been seen before. In 1871, Dr. Cassandra Durham of Plains was heralded as the first female doctor in the state of Georgia, a status that Dr. Durham achieved with difficulty but which earned her respect in her lifetime and after it.[3] Nursing was the best compromise for a young woman of good family, and Lillian knew the only way she could get her father to agree to her training was to appeal to the patriotism sweeping the nation at war. In 1917, she finally received Jim Jack's assent. She mailed in her application and dreamed of the day when she could finally begin her training.

She didn't know it yet, but in those weeks waiting for a response to her application, Lillian would find herself in the role she so desired, but in circumstances she would look back on with pain.

Starting in June 1918, a virulent strain of Spanish influenza began to spread so rapidly it had circled the globe within a year, leaving no country untouched. It killed mostly the young and healthy, and was nearly always fatal, causing a panic worldwide. Annie Lee Gordy, Lillian's next eldest sister, was born in 1894, and had married Jay G. Webb, by whom she was pregnant with their first child. Both Jay and Annie fell sick with the flu, and as timing would have it, there were no other family members to look after them except for Lillian. "My mother was going through the change of life," she explained, "and my other sister had a teeny baby. I was the only one who could go in the house." By this time, Lillian was already a caregiver within the family. With so many children to look after, Ida couldn't do it all; Lillian took care of her younger siblings, as remembered by her sister Elizabeth. "Sometimes when she's tired," she remembered, "she limps a little bit, and she says that's because she had to carry me around for a year or so." She bore the load again at the bedsides of her sister and brother-in-law. Perhaps because Jay was a few years older, and certainly because he wasn't carrying a baby, Annie's husband pulled through. But Lillian could only watch as her sister sank rapidly. Annie and her unborn child died on November 11, 1918, the same day the armistice was signed between the victorious allies and defeated Germany and the same day, with an irony Lillian never forgot, that acceptance of her application for nurse's training arrived in the mail. "My sister's death caused me great agony," she said later. But her care for Annie Lee during her illness, and the acceptance letter from the government, strengthened her determination and her case that a nursing career was what she was born for. "I thought," she recalled for an interview years later, "'Oh, how I would like to spend my life doing something like this.'"[4]

In the Georgia of 1920, the year Lillian left home to pursue her training, Grady Memorial Hospital in Atlanta was the most important medical center in the state. It was however a place to complete one's training, not begin it. Luckily for Lillian, she was able to have her beginning as nurse not all that far from Richland—in Plains, a small town with the distinction of being named for a singularly violent and miraculous test of faith.

Plains was originally called Plains of Dura, after the place in the Book of Daniel where King Nebuchadnezzar consigns the Israelites Shadrach, Meshach and Abednego to a fiery furnace for refusing to worship his golden idol.[5] The town's topography also helped suggest its name. Save for where fields of cotton and peanuts press the land more or less flat, as by a hand smoothing a quilt, that same coverlet lay rucked and rumpled elsewhere, its ridges studded with the stockades of skinny Georgia pines. Plains lay among these folds of red dirt fields, pinned to the map by its water tower and the fact that a train stopped there, shaping the community that developed around it. In the nineteenth century, a small town's survival depended on proximity to rail transport, which is why so many hamlets were strung throughout the United States like weathered beads on steel string, much as the same is true now for big box and fast-food towns adjacent to modern highways. When a line was laid from Americus, the bustling Sumter County seat a little over ten miles to the east of Plains, it ran close but not close enough to the original location of Plains, so the town fathers moved the town to the rails, and built a long, low white wooden depot alongside the gleaming tracks. If Richland's layout spoke to order and hierarchy, Plains' was shaped by the bulky edifice of businesses joined along its central street, like a well-laden trawler being pulled by the tugboat of the train depot. Until 1929, these shops and warehouses and dusty roads bustled with the prosperity not just of cotton but of peanuts, which had been introduced to the area only a decade before Lillian's arrival. This made for the sort of place where white gingerbread houses loomed above the trees, their porches refuges of cool hospitality on warm summer evenings, lemonade or sweet tea or something stronger passed from black hands to white ones. That it was also a devout place could be seen in its churches, especially Plains Baptist, its rich stained glass windows and crisp Gothic arches proclaiming the value of both worldly and spiritual goods, at least for the white people who worshipped there.

Plains was mobbed by the outside world when Jimmy Carter announced his candidacy for president of the United States, and to a degree though the crowds are nowhere near as bountiful as they were in 1976–80, the presence of Jimmy and Rosalynn Carter still brings people there. What has not changed, though, from the first days of the town's existence, are all the grace notes of this place that Lillian Carter preferred to any other on earth: the straight-backed pines, the snowy dollops of cotton and the little russet hills of turned peanuts; the pink and purple sunsets and the way night falls impenetrably dark as dreamless sleep; the fluting of doves in the morning. Beneath these surface qualities, then as now, was a special, unique something which flows through Plains like a slow, silent southern river, a quiet music you can never hear if you're just passing through. When Lillian insisted she disliked cities and was really a "country person" at heart, she didn't mean just any old country setting. She meant Plains, for all of the above reasons and plenty that even a Plains native cannot define. It was in this place of good clean commerce and good clean religion (or what appeared to be the case) that the Wise brothers founded the hospital that attracted Lillian to the next chapter of her destiny.

Established in Plains in 1912, the Wise Sanitarium was no rustic affair. It was a fully equipped hospital created and staffed by Doctors Samuel, Thaddeus and Bowman Wise, sons of Dr. Burr T. Wise, a South Carolinian of German descent who had become a prominent member of the Plains community. The Sanitarium that Lillian first knew was a twenty bed clinic

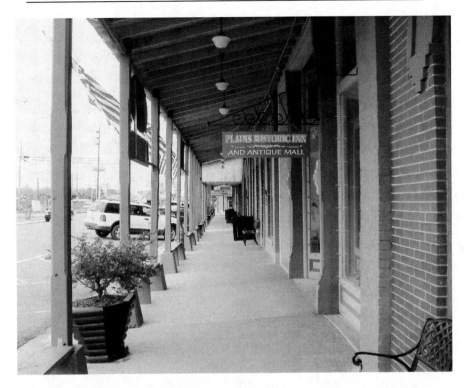

A view down Main Street, Plains, Georgia. There is a special, unique something which flows through Plains like a slow, silent southern river, a quiet music you can never hear if you're just passing through (photograph by the author).

situated on the second floor of a building along the Main Street of Plains; in 1921 it would be established in its own building, a Greek Revival structure still extant on the outskirts of the town (now the Lillian G. Carter Nursing Home). Among its distinctions, the Wise Sanitarium was one of the first small hospitals in America to be granted accreditation by the American College of Surgeons and the American Medical and Hospital Association.[6]

As a training hospital, the Wise Sanitarium pulled no punches. Years later, Lillian would describe how from the first day of her training she was challenged by successive difficulties, to be overcome while simultaneously caring for patients in increasing degrees of responsibility. There were more mundane chores as well. While it was inconvenient to go up and down the stairs of the two story building so many times each day, it at least broke up the constant standing on hard floors required of a nurse on duty. Lillian remembered how much more disagreeable these stairs became when the girls had to carry heavy or unwieldy items. This included containers of waste material that would normally have been flushed down a drain or toilet, a job which nowadays is the responsibility of orderlies. "We had to empty bed pans in a barrel," she explained in one example, "and carry it down," taking great care not to spill the contents. The young trainees also had to contend with another challenge, the "tough" head nurse, who came from Grady Hospital in Atlanta and was a lady for whom no-nonsense was a religion. This nurse, Mrs. Gussie Abrams, was to prove to possess a soft center and would become an ally of Lillian's in the coming years. She was also something of an anomaly in straight-laced Plains: though still married to Mr. Abrams, she was living with one of the Wise brothers, Dr. Thad, and even bore him a child which, as Jimmy Carter relates, died young and was buried in the Abrams family plot.[7] Regardless of her unconventional personal life, Mrs. Abrams didn't hesitate to lay down the law with her girls. "We were restricted if we did the least little thing out of place," Lillian remembered. For some infraction she doesn't describe, she was once refused permission to have a date for a week. "We were never allowed to go out at night," she added, "except on the weekends."[8]

There were other demands of a patient-related nature. One case gives a sense of the sort of sophisticated procedures that the Wise Sanitarium, though in the middle of rural Georgia, was comfortable carrying out. It also shows what sort of prudence and composure was required of a young and relatively inexperienced nurse. An elderly man whom Lillian knew as a neighbor had had a prostatectomy, a surgery that had first been achieved in England in the late 1880s to treat enlarged prostate. The patient had to be watched because he kept trying to pull out the catheter, and it was Lillian's job to make sure he didn't do so. Those were the days before efficient and regulated tranquilizers and painkillers. In pain and likely emotionally upset as well, the man waited till Lillian turned her back and pulled out the tube. Lillian's recollection of the incident makes it sound as if she had never had to perform this sort of intimate procedure before, which given her inexperience is probably true. Even so, conducting herself like a professional, Lillian got the catheter back in and made sure it stayed there, even if it meant spending the entire night with one eye on her patient. As a young nurse, "that was the worst experience I ever had," Lillian confided later. It was a specifically male problem for a woman to deal with and one which would reappear in her life again many decades later in a family planning clinic in India.[9]

Conditions improved once the Wises moved to their new hospital. The sixty beds were all on one floor, leaving stairs behind for good, and the space offered a proper operating room as well as an x-ray room where radium treatments could be given. This was where most of Lillian's training took place, and it was here she began to lose her fear of the Wise doctors. The trust was mutual. Shortly after the move to the new facility, the Wises hired a nurse specifically for the operating room. Lillian was put to work there assisting her. "In about two months," she recalled, "they let the operating nurse go, and I had the operating room as my own for the rest of the time." At the Wise Sanitarium, the operating room nurse was no sponge assistant or general gofer. "I assisted the doctors," Lillian carefully explained.[10] When writing his 2004 memoir of his mother, Jimmy Carter consulted her 1921 *Lippincott's Nursing Manual*, a small volume nicked and worn from being thumbed, carried and consulted through countless visits. With this book and the knowledge she had picked up through hands-on training, Lillian had prepared herself for the state board exam. In the manual she inscribed her name, "Miss Lillian Gordy," nine times (perhaps because she had often had to lend it to fellow nurses, and wanted to make sure it came back), and listed all the nurses in training for the year 1922. What struck Carter was the fact that the entry dealing with syphilis was boldly underscored.[11] Sexually transmitted disease was believed by most white laymen as well as doctors to be specially endemic in black people, the result of the sin of presumed promiscuity. "Syphilitic complications were widely considered to be influenced by race (ie, neurosyphilis more common in whites, cardiovascular disease more common in blacks, and overall complications more common in whites than in blacks)," write the authors of a 2004 article on the execrable United States Public Health study of the effects of untreated syphilis on black men. The Tuskegee Study of Untreated Syphilis, or TSUS as it became known, was carried out in Tuskegee, Alabama from 1932 until well past the administration of President John F. Kennedy. "Some studies of the day suggested that syphilis did not always need to be treated—that it could often remain quiescent, especially in blacks," state the article's authors. Even after penicillin was approved for broad use after World War II, it wasn't given to these men, whose symptoms were watched with interest in the experiment but a disinterest in the rights and the human dignity of the men, which seemed to symbolize the way the health issues of blacks were treated by many whites of the day, in and out of the south.[12] As W.E. B. Dubois put it acidly and succinctly, "While sociologists gleefully count his bastards and his prostitutes, the very soul of the toiling, sweating black man is darkened by the shadow of a vast despair."[13]

Perusing his mother's nursing manual, Jimmy Carter noticed something else, related in a way to the syphilis issue—that the book dealt with so many illnesses which few people in twenty-first century America have ever heard of, let alone experienced, "most of them now of concern only to people in Africa and a few other places in the Third World." (The eradication of illnesses even more medieval than these, such as dracunculiasis, lymphatic filariasis, and cysticercosis, would become the intense focus of The Carter Center's pioneering programs in Africa.)[14]

The south had been that Third World for many of the blacks who lived around Plains, which lay in the center of the so-called Black Belt of Georgia, before the Civil War and for too long after it. As late as 1940, the black death rate from pulmonary diseases like influenza and pneumonia was three times greater than that of white. Black babies had half the chance of white ones in surviving the many diseases infants and children were exposed to.[15] As Jimmy Carter knew too well from having survived childhood in an era when diseases now treatable were a real threat even to healthy children, the rural setting of Plains might have been a safe place to cross the street unaided but not to avoid dire sickness. In the early 1930s, he found, nearly half of rural schoolchildren were infected with hookworm, a consequence of running barefoot (often because of lack of shoes) and living without proper hygiene, two attributes of the poor. Once established in the intestines, hookworm robbed its host of whatever nutrients the body took in, which for a child of the poor often was little enough to begin with. The treatment for many of what we would now consider the most dangerous illnesses was not much more advanced than taking aspirin (if you had it), or rubbing on some Mercurochrome, or something Carter remembered called "666 Cold Preparation," "and various patent medicines that were primarily alcohol," Carter wrote, "and sometimes opium." To ward off winter illnesses children were sent to school wearing bags around their neck filled with foul-smelling asafetida root. A white person's childhood in the first decades of the twentieth century was a world where if a remedy stank or stung, it was all the more healing. If this world was a dangerous place for middle class folks like the Carters, it was many times more so for impoverished black families whose illnesses or injuries went untreated, for whom even Mercurochrome was a luxury few could afford.[16]

Not far from Plains was a resort called Magnolia Springs, first described in a June 1858 edition of the *Americus Times-Recorder* as "Sumter Mineral Springs ... a general place of resort for the young folks and everybody in general," with a hotel and "bathing house" on the premises. Over sixty years later, long after the days of hoopskirts and slaves, for those living in Plains, Magnolia Springs was still about the only respectable place an unmarried young man and woman could go to relax away from the eyes of elders. Before Lillian's training at the Sanitarium officially began, she went out to Magnolia Springs one Sunday night for some fun. "I had a date with a boy named George Tanner," Lillian remembered. He was a burly man, large-framed, who worked for a local sawmill, and probably wouldn't have been allowed in her parents' front yard, let alone the front parlor, had Lillian had the temerity to bring him home to Richland. But she liked George, who had a nice sister, Lucy. That night, Lucy brought her own date, a young man named James Earl Carter. A grocer, something of a ladies man, and inveterate poker player (if the nurses at the Sanitarium were to be believed), and wearing spectacles, Carter was already known to Lillian, and she did not like him.[17] She had seen him in the resort pool, "ostentatiously doing front flips and half gainers off the springboard into the frigid water," as Lillian told son Jimmy.[18] She thought of Carter as a showoff who considered himself too clever by half, and when she discovered that he was Lucy's date she was not amused. As if to show her how little her opinion of him mattered, Lillian remembered, Carter spent the entire evening without asking her to dance, though he did so once when suggested by George Tanner—for a pretty and popular southern girl, this was the insult of all insults. Lillian remained unmoved. "I couldn't stand him," she recalled.[19]

Dr. Sam Wise was impressed by Lillian's innate skill and quick intelligence, and made a practice of looking out for her. "When I was going with George," she said, "he didn't like it at all." Dr. Sam was not only a friend of Jim Jack's but a friend of Earl Carter's, which may have emboldened him to take on the role of father figure and, not surprisingly, that of Cupid. (Like many of Nature's born matchmakers, Dr. Sam was not married and contented himself by dating the prettiest nurses, according to Jimmy Carter—a prosthetic leg, the result of a childhood disease, never kept him from capering with them on the dance floor.) Dr. Sam told Lillian he didn't approve of George Tanner, and that he had already picked out someone for her in Plains "who is going to be the most successful man here, and that's Earl Carter."[20] Carter certainly came of respectable if occasionally bloody background. Born in Arlington, a little over fifty miles south from Plains, on September 12, 1894, he was a great-grandson of Wiley Carter, first of the family to be born in Georgia. By his death in 1864 Wiley had amassed a plantation of over two thousand acres, with "two graceful two story houses" and 150 slaves in Schley County. Though married to gentle women, including Earl's South Carolinian mother, Nina Pratt, some of the hard edges of these vigorous Carter men had only been blunted rather than smoothed. For three generations, death by gun was to haunt the Carters: Wiley Carter killed a man over disputed ownership of a slave; his son Littleberry was himself killed in an argument over a "flying jenny," a primitive form of carnival merry-go-round; and his son, William Archibald, father of Earl, was shot and killed in 1903 in an altercation with a tenant. Thus Earl was made fatherless at the age of nine, a factor which likely shaped his cautious and conservative approach to life later on. It probably also contributed to his need to show off at the Magnolia Springs pool and devote an evening every week to a card game the focus of which was what kind of hand Fate dealt your opponent and what kind of hand she decided to deal to you.[21]

A week after her single dance with Earl, Lillian was in the Plains drugstore, which occupied the space under the trainees' dorm, with some of her friends from the training program when Earl approached her—he had been outside with friends, clearly waiting for her to pass by. He tipped his hat, wished her good morning, and told her how happy he was to see her again. He then asked her if she would take a ride with him that weekend. "He had a car," Lillian remembered. "It was a little Model T without a top." His courtly manner, so different from the Earl Carter whose swimming pool antics had made her sneer, won the day. She agreed to ride with him.[22]

Lillian would point out that though she made Earl come up to the front door of the trainees' dormitory to fetch her that weekend, as any gentleman should (and no doubt as Gussie Abrams would have insisted), she couldn't resist peeking at him from the balcony, more excited than she expected to be. She'd gone to the trouble of borrowing a blue silk dress from another nurse, who lent it out regularly for similar special occasions, so she was obviously recovered from her attitude of studied indifference. Earl handed her into his car, cranked the engine, and off they went. "It was a little before sundown," Lillian explained to Jimmy Carter, "and he said he was going to drive out toward Preston and show me the farmland his family owned. I reckon he wanted to make an impression regarding how well-off they were." But the drive, as it happened, didn't go as planned. "We hadn't got to Choctahatchee Creek," she went on, "before it started pouring down rain." Like a scene from one of the romantic comedies then all the rage on the silent screen, in which improbable lovers are thrown together by a storm, Earl and Lillian each took a corner of the car's lap robe and held it over their heads as Earl drove the car across a field to the refuge of a wagon shed on his family's property. There they sat until the downpour stopped.[23]

As Lillian later told her eldest son, when it was dry enough for them to get the car started and leave, "we were pretty well acquainted by the time we got back to town." (She would later qualify that account by insisting she had not allowed Earl to kiss her until they had been courting a couple of months.)[24] They had a proper first date soon after the wagon shed adventure, when Earl took Lillian to Americus to see a production of *The Merchant of Venice*. As she would Ruth and Esther, those two strong and influential women in the Bible, Lillian admired the character of Portia, whose intelligence and courage save a life and bring her the love she desires. Like the play's heroine, Lillian not only loved to match wits with any man but to demonstrate the quality and the uses of mercy: "It blesseth him that gives," Portia says, "and him that takes."[25]

It was an evening some might think more literary than romantic, but not for Lillian, and probably not for Earl. Though the latter, according to Jimmy Carter, in later life mostly read the newspaper or farming journals, he had a respectable small library of books that he had clearly read, as they were signed and numbered by him. One of these was *Royal Road to Romance* by handsome and daring Princeton graduate (and Tennessee boy) Richard Halliburton, the color and fantasy of whose brief life—and perhaps some of the dreams of young Earl Carter—can be seen in its opening chapter:

> I hungered for the romance of great mountains. From childhood I had dreamed of climbing Fujiyama and the Matterhorn, and had planned to charge Mount Olympus in order to visit the gods that dwelled there. I wanted to swim the Hellespont ... float down the Nile in a butterfly boat, make love to a pale Kashmiri maiden beside the Shalimar, dance to the castanets of Granada gypsies, commune in solitude with the moonlit Taj Mahal, hunt tigers in a Bengal jungle—try everything once.[26]

This was romance that Lillian could well appreciate, and love.

She also quickly learned to appreciate Earl's more workaday gifts, what she called his get up and go. He had not had as much education as she—he had attended Riverside Military Academy, located near Gainesville, Georgia in the foothills of the Blue Ridge Mountains, only until the tenth grade—but his innate intelligence and his almost supernatural understanding of what plus what would equal profits impressed everyone, including her. On leaving school, he had enlisted in the army, serving the Quartermaster Corps as a first lieutenant during World War I. As it turned out, this was a valuable education unto itself, as the Corps specialized in supply and distribution, talent for which Earl was to demonstrate during his future business career. As Hugh Carter, Earl's nephew, put it, it seemed that anything Earl Carter touched turned to gold.[27]

Lillian explained in an interview years later, "He worked for his brother [Alton] in a grocery ... he also had a pressing club.... It's where you take clothes to be cleaned. In those days a Negro man did the cleaning and pressing. He also had the ice house, where you sold ice by fifty pounds or a hundred." Besides these business interests, Earl had bought a farm of some four hundred acres, which Lillian remembered had cost him $7,000. "That's the last thing he ever bought on credit," she pointed out. Not, she added, that Earl was the sort of farmer with dirt under his fingernails. "He loved farming," she recalled, to such a degree that she once joked with him, "Lord, honey, if you were to die you'd have to go by the farm first." Yet he never plowed an acre of it himself. "He never did anything," she said matter of factly. "He had blacks to do that."[28]

After they had been seeing one another for some time, Earl became a familiar figure in the little parlor of the nurse trainees' dormitory; he even became a favorite, according to Lillian, of Gussie Abrams, who let him enter the place at will. Earl was sitting in the parlor one day waiting for Lillian when she walked in to find him looking "heartbroken" and "really mad." His sixteen year old sister Jeannette had eloped and married in secret. Earl blurted out: "I had so wanted us to be married before she did, but now I've got to look after her." Lillian was far more interested in what he had said about marrying *her*: it was the first time he had ever broached the subject openly. Then he said something else. "I want you to finish training," he said, "and then we'll get married." When she had completed her training, he told her, "you'll always have something to fall back on." If Lillian was thrilled to hear the part about getting married, it was because her pursuit of her chosen career had proved to be so wearying. "I got tired of training," she said later. "It was hard work." But Earl was clearly not going to be some run of the mill chauvinist, happy to have the little woman in the kitchen, forever pregnant and dependent. After all, American (white) women had finally received the vote in 1920; it was high time they went after the careers they had fought to get. Earl's resolve and his promise kept Lillian at her work at the Sanitarium, as it did later in Atlanta, where she went for six months to train at Grady Hospital in the specialized areas of women's and children's diseases.[29]

Atlanta was a world away from Plains, and Lillian missed Earl very much. "You had to get on a train," she recalled, "and ride all day and half the night getting back." Earl came to see her twice while she was there, and he telephoned her every Sunday, so she wasn't utterly bereft. It was at Grady Hospital that she received her engagement ring from him—through the mail. One of the interns, a Doctor Ridley, was a friend of Lillian's and offered to pick up her mail, as the strict nursing schedule allowed her few opportunities to get it herself. Ridley, she remembered, "had slipped the letter in his pocket in a little package, and that was my ring." Many women might not be so thrilled to receive this next to most important ring via the United States postal service, but Lillian was ecstatic. "It was terrific," she recalled.[30]

Also terrific was the reception Earl received from the Gordys in Richland. "My people were crazy about him," Lillian said. "They knew he was good, and he was going to be successful, and he was everything they had wanted for me."[31] Not that the Gordys didn't take some getting used to for Earl. Earl's family never gathered for Sunday dinner, as Jimmy Carter recalled, but when the Gordys got together they usually argued—on many a drive over to Richland, Earl and Lillian would amusedly try to guess what subject would command the field of the dinner table that particular Sunday. He would also never understand the Gordy habit of reading at the dinner table. Because of his poor eyesight, and by choice, Earl was not an inveterate reader (his business interests left him with little time for anything else) and at future family suppers would find himself the sole member of his household without a book in one hand and a fork in the other.[32] He was, however, clearly lovable, an attribute no Gordy ever took for granted. Emily Gordy Dolvin was especially fond of Earl, as she recalled years later. After Lillian and Earl married, Emily would spend her summers in Plains, to help Lillian look after her growing family. "I used to ride with Earl over the Webster County farms in his pickup truck," she said, "ride over the cotton fields and all around with Earl. He loved me and I loved him." When she left for Georgia State College for Women in Millidgeville, she remembered, Earl gave her $75 to take with her. "That was just a lot of money for the day," she explained. But he gave it to her, she said, "because he loved me."[33]

None of Lillian's family was present for the marriage ceremony that took place in Plains on Thursday, September 27, 1923. "We were not going to have a wedding," Lillian explained. "At that time my family—we were not able to have a big wedding. We were just going to marry quietly at the minister's house." That they did, with one other couple who were also getting married, and with Gussie Abrams in attendance. A trip to Atlanta afterward had been planned by the newlyweds, but an embarrassing problem arose that prevented them from taking the two hour train ride—namely, Lillian had a boil on her bottom which made sitting excruciating. So their first night was spent in the house of Nina Pratt Carter, after which they moved into a room in the Wellons' boarding house on Church Street, a tall, handsome Georgian Revival place with balconied gables and colored glass windows across the railroad tracks from the business block and Lillian's former domicile over the drugstore. The room was furnished through Earl's purchase of some furniture and the numerous presents the couple had been given for their wedding. They were to get to know this room quite well in the first weeks, because as it happened, like the trip to Atlanta, the Carters' honeymoon was also postponed. "When we were going to get married," Lillian remembered, "[Earl] had planted a lot of Irish potatoes [on his farm]. He said, 'When we sell those potatoes, that's when we'll go on our honeymoon.' The potatoes were a flop!"[34]

What Lillian wanted most, though, was something closer to home—to get pregnant, "so they wouldn't call me on duty." Earl had sped up the process of her certification by talking to the officials at Grady Hospital, who agreed to waive the waiting period and allow Lillian to take her state board examination immediately. As a result, Wise Sanitarium had one of their best new nurses suddenly at their beck and call, and beck and call they did. Dr. Sam Wise would ask Lillian, "Please do this. We need you so bad." And so she went on duty several times a week. "Earl was willing," she remembered, "as long as I didn't have to do night duty," a remarkable degree of latitude from a young husband just two decades into the twentieth century.[35]

Life with her new husband was not the smooth ride Lillian may have hoped (nor, to be fair, was it likely so for Earl). As Lillian told her eldest son, she suddenly found herself living with a man who wouldn't put off all his bachelor ways. "He told me before we were married that he played poker every Friday night," she said to Jimmy, "but I figured I could break him of that. The first Friday after we were married he left right after supper and came home long after midnight. I refused to speak to him and pouted for a day or so, but it didn't do any good—then or later." Earl's nature was so generous, Lillian said, that it spilled over, often not in her direction. On just one occasion, when she was pregnant a friend delighted her by sending over some grapes to help her through a patch of nausea. But on seeing them, Earl thought immediately of Ethel Wellons, member of the family in whose house the Carters had their first apartment. She was pregnant, too, and Earl had heard she was also not feeling well. "I'd like to take the grapes to her," he told his wife. Lillian was furious, and in a southern belle pique, "I threw them at him."[36]

Earl tended to operate on principles of good sense rather than romantic ardor when choosing gifts for Lillian. "That first Christmas," she recalled, "he went over to Plains Mercantile Co. at the last minute and bought me a lap robe. I was really mad that he didn't get me something more nice and personal." And the large diamond he was to give her for a ring she wore till her death was not selected from a jeweler's window but obtained at discount from the Baptist church after an anonymous tither left it in the collection plate. Still, his sheer largesse could astonish her. When they were still engaged, Earl had given Lillian a purse containing three coins—thirty-five dollars, in gold. "It was the most money I had ever had at one time," she remembered. Even the unfortunate fact that someone in the trainees' dormitory stole the money didn't lessen the gift's significance for Lillian.[37]

Lillian had married a man who, as she would discover—and continue discovering—was not what or who he seemed. Many people then and now saw what they wanted to see in Earl Carter: a hard-nosed businessman, an unrepentant segregationist, a man incapable of dreaming the big dreams that for Lillian Carter were the reason for living. Yet Lillian looked deeper into Earl's nature than anyone else could. "We had different ways," Lillian explained to Jimmy years later, "and it took us a long time to figure out how much room to give each other."[38] For all their differences, they clicked. Nearly a quarter century after Earl's death, she would still tell friends, "I have never ceased being lonely for him, but I've never been lonely for anyone else."[39]

CHAPTER 3

Nurse and Mother

The Wellons house still stands on Church Street in Plains. At the top of its two mahogany staircases is a door with a plaque beside it stating that it was here that James Earl Carter and Lillian Gordy Carter lived in 1924, "when Mrs. Carter was expecting the future president." On the door, over the brass "2," is another, smaller sign, also of brass but engraved with lettering whose fluted dignity belies the humorous message it conveys: "The Conception Room." Whether or not this was actually the place where the thirty-ninth President of the United States was conceived (local lore has it that the conception occurred under a pecan tree, the exact location of which is a state secret), Lillian assured her son in later years that "that room is where we first learned that you would be born."[1]

The catalyst in bringing Lillian and Earl together, Dr. Sam also played a part in deciding their domestic living arrangements. The Carters had remained at the Wellons house "until Dr. Sam Wise said I couldn't go up and down the stairs anymore," Lillian told Jimmy. So on doctor's orders, Earl and Lillian moved to the ground floor of another house in Plains that was owned by Emmett and Bessie Cook. In the meantime, Dr. Sam encouraged Lillian to keep working as long as she felt she could, advice that was as unheard-of in those times, when pregnant women often remained secluded as soon as they "started showing," as it is commonplace today.[2]

Lillian's maternity would have about it another innovation for the era and locale. Most babies in or around Plains were born at home, ushered in by a midwife or an experienced elder female of the family, or sometimes a country doctor. While the father paced nervously in the parlor or worked outside to make the time pass, water would be put on the stove to boil, and women with the same knowing expression prepared clean rags, scissors and twine. It was not just Lillian's decision to change that age-old pattern but Dr. Sam's. His offer of a room at Wise Sanitarium "made me the answer to a Trivial Pursuit question," Jimmy Carter wryly pointed out in later years: "'Who was the first U.S. president to be born in a hospital?'"[3]

The last day of September 1924, around 10 o'clock in the evening, Lillian began to feel the first serious pains, and Earl, a stickler for schedules and preparedness, said "Let's get ready quick." But as Lillian jokingly told an interviewer in later years, she replied to her husband, "I'm not going until I take a bath." An hour later, they were met at the hospital by Dr. Sam; and a little before sunrise, "at exactly 7 o'clock in the morning," Lillian recalled, "Jimmy was born." Lillian awoke from the ether to a jubilant Earl, glowing and grinning at having sired a son, whom he and Lillian named James Earl Carter, Jr. "He was just so happy, he didn't know what to do," she said. Earl now had a boy to carry on the family name, and on whom he could project the ideals of intelligence and endurance that powered all his own activities, as businessman and private person. As would be seen years later, when youngest and last child Billy was born, where Billy was indulged Jimmy was made to earn everything he had, including paternal approval he never quite felt he achieved. Thus his childhood would be suffused with an atmosphere of noblesse oblige. There are those to whom much has been given, Jimmy was taught in the cradle, and there are those to whom you owed service because nothing had been given to them at all.[4]

The Carters were not long for the Cooks'. The dog that some well-wishing friend brought over as a gift for infant Jimmy was apparently the last straw for Bessie Cook; she objected so vociferously that the only recourse for the Carters was to move. Earl was doing well enough to do more than rent, so he and Lillian bought a house on Bond Street, next door to the broad-porched bungalow of the Smiths, Edgar and Allie. In the Smith house in 1927 a child would be born, a girl named Eleanor Rosalynn, who was to play a role in Jimmy Carter's life beyond the imaginings of the Smiths or the Carters.[5]

Not long after the family moved to Bond Street, and shortly before the birth of their first daughter, Gloria, they came close to losing two-year-old Jimmy. He fell sick with colitis, the inflammation of the colon that through loss of blood and fluids proved deadly to both children and adults. That Lillian was several months pregnant may indicate that Jimmy's illness was an inadvertent consequence of his being weaned off his mother's milk.

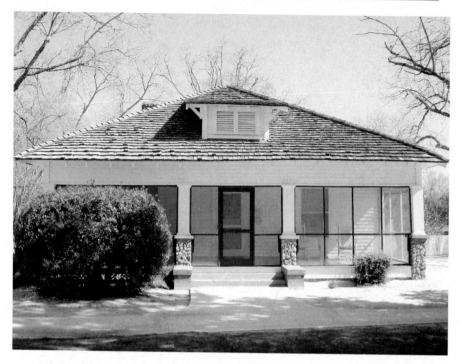

The Carter farm, located between Plains and Archery. A basic house by any standard, it nevertheless boasted amenities enjoyed by few in the surrounding region, particularly during the Great Depression (photograph by the author).

Lillian and Earl brought Jimmy to the Sanitarium, where a specialist came from Macon to examine and treat him. He didn't improve. Lillian had been acquainted with a country doctor from the town of Montezuma, east of Plains, and had worked with him during operations at the Sanitarium. Something moved her to appeal to him, and the doctor examined the child. "He said, 'If you'll do what I say, I can cure him,'" Lillian told an interviewer years later. The remedy sounds deceptively simple: saturated solution of cornstarch administered in the rectum via slow-drip enema, which coated the colon and prevented further irritation, allowing the tissues to heal. Jimmy's was not the only life Lillian would save with the cornstarch miracle. Over the years, whenever there was a case of colitis, Dr. Sam would call Lillian and say, "'Would you go do that?'"[6]

      As with Mrs. Cook's house, the Carters' residence on Bond Street was also brief. In 1928, Lillian and Earl traded the house for a farm located nearly three miles west of Plains, just the other side of the border between Sumter and Webster counties. Part of this decision was because the Carters needed a home that could accommodate their growing family. But it was also something of a businessman's canny investment and of something else, less tangible but even stronger. Earl was eager to derive profit from his every undertaking, yet he also seemed to want the land for another reason: like the plantation lost to his ancestors in the Civil War, a farm would allow him to be self-sufficient. "Daddy didn't believe in paying for something that we could do ourselves," Jimmy Carter wrote. Like some of the larger antebellum plantations, the place would even boast a commissary, stocked with items from the store Earl had run in Plains, so that his tenants and others living outside town could purchase essentials, oil for light and heat, matches, dry goods, even clothes and shoes, to be charged against their Saturday paydays. In the next decade, Earl's preference for being on the distributing rather than receiving end of any transaction would run up against what he and other southern farmers saw as the invasive New Deal policies of President Franklin D. Roosevelt (whom Lillian, disregarding her husband's political beliefs, defiantly admired and voted for).[7]

Earl chose his acreage wisely. Jimmy Carter remembered that his father's farm comprised what remained of good farmland so far west, and the soil was rich enough to bear all the demands Earl put on it. It became a pervasive substance of Jimmy Carter's childhood. Since Highway 208 passed in front of the house, parallel to the tracks of the Seaboard Airline Railroad, there was a continual cloud of terracotta dust, when it wasn't raining. Carter commemorated it in his memoirs:

> My most persistent impression as a farm boy was of the earth. There was a closeness, almost an immersion, in the sand, loam, and red clay that seemed natural, and constant. The soil caressed my bare feet, and the dust was always boiling up from the dirt road that passed fifty feet from our door, so that inside our clapboard house the red clay particles, ranging in size from face powder to grits, were ever present.[8]

The three bedroom house, a single story bungalow painted tan, with screened porches fore and aft and a steeply pitched roof to ward off the summer sun, had been built by a local family using plans obtained from Sears, Roebuck and Company, whose fantastically diverse catalog children were known to search for a way to order a pony. Sears had offered house plans since early in the century, bringing out a series of "kit-houses" in which all the parts and pieces, numbered for assembly, were shipped to clients to be put together on their lot.[9] The Carters' house was a compact, serviceable yet comfortable dwelling. Off the central hall were the bedrooms (and later a bathroom) on one side and dining room, kitchen and breakfast room on the other, with high glass windows and smooth plank

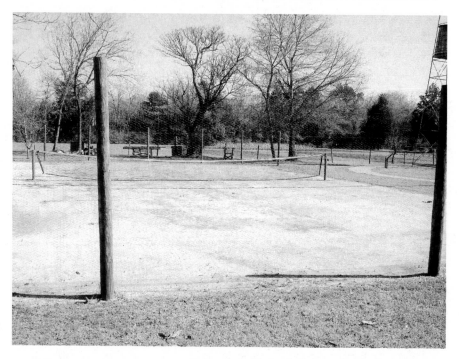

The tennis court on the Carter farm, which was anything but hardscrabble (photograph by the author).

floors, and spare but handsome moldings. Like the house itself, the clean, simple, square furniture inside it all spoke to a frugality and a no-frills atmosphere, even as the upright Baldwin piano and the shelves of books—Twain, Dickinson, Eliot, Chaucer, Dickens—spoke to the richer realm of the mind and spirit which Lillian and Earl were able to offer their children. As Lillian would tell interviewer Mike Douglas in December 1976, "We spent more money on books than we did on clothes!" The house didn't have running water until 1935 or electric light till three years after that, but compared to the cabins of the tenants, where newspapers lined the bare wood walls of rooms shadowed in stove soot and where the occupants could see the ground through cracks in the floor (if they had one), it was a veritable mansion.[10]

The year after they moved in, two months before the stock market crash, Lillian gave birth to another daughter, Ruth, whose blonde curls and winsome ways soon had Earl wrapped around her little finger. "Gloria and I learned quite early how best to deal with Daddy and Mama," recalled Jimmy Carter. "He was a stern but fair disciplinarian, whose word was absolute law in our house." Lillian could be appealed to through confession of any misdeeds; if one of her lukewarm spankings resulted, she always said as much to Earl, telling him, "I've already punished them." Compared to the switch he used on their legs, Lillian's method was far preferred.[11]

Lillian admitted she was not the most demonstrative of mothers. "[Earl] was a more affectionate father than I was a mother," she said. Perhaps losing his father so young sensitized him to the emotional needs of his own children and underscored the importance of family togetherness. "Every night the children would go to their daddy," recalled Lillian, "and kneel down beside him to say their prayers."[12] It was Earl who read stories to the children. Yet Lillian, for all that she had a detached, almost professional attitude toward her brood, had a talent for bringing magic into their lives. "Christmas was a time of enchantment for the Carter family," Lillian wrote. "Everything had a breathless expectancy about it." Hunting for a Christmas tree with Earl and decorating it with their mother was just part of what thrilled the children during the holidays. There were also visits with her to the homes of poor families, to whom the children gave baskets of food and clothing. "It was a magic time for all," Lillian recalled. Such was not the mood at Christmas 1934, however. All the Carter children came down with the measles. "Instead of baking cookies and preparing for our traditional Christmas breakfast and dinner," wrote Lillian, "I spent my time bathing feverish little foreheads, easing sore throats and soothing pain-filled eyes." The children's beds were moved into one bedroom to make it easier for Lillian to take care of them, and it was while they lay prone that Earl read to them Luke's account of the nativity from the Bible. "Wan white faces looked bleakly up from their pillows," Lillian remembered. Watching Earl put together the children's toys—their first bicycles, which they wouldn't be well enough to ride for weeks after Christmas—Lillian wept as Christmas tunes were broadcast over the radio on WSB out of Atlanta. "Then I heard the announcer tell about Little Jack Little," she said, "a nationally famous radio and vaudeville personality of that day." Little was in Atlanta and would be singing over the station for Christmas Day. Early Christmas morning, Lillian gamely dialed through to WSB, and Little Jack Little came on the phone to hear her request. "Let me see what I can do," he told her. Later, Lillian roused the children, telling them she thought they'd like to hear some carols. "Little Jack Little came on singing Christmas tunes and thumping the piano," she recalled; too sick to care, Jimmy, Gloria and Ruth lay quietly listening. Just before the program ended, Little made an announcement: "And now I'm going to sing a song especially for three little Carter children who are ill: Jimmy, Ruth and Gloria." As "three little heads jerked up," Lillian recalled, Jack Little sang a comic song the children loved, Lou Handman's "Wooden Head, Puddin' Head Jones." When the sore-throated children tried to sing along, Lillian and Earl stood at the door to listen, tears streaming. "Thanks to someone who had room in his heart to listen to a farm wife's plea," Lillian wrote, "it turned out to be one of the most memorable Christmases we ever had." True to the uniqueness of Lillian's household, "Wooden Head, Puddin' Head Jones" became a most unlikely and beloved Christmas carol in the Carter family.[13]

"They had a good home life," Lillian said of her children, "and lived with a father and mother daily who are more or less Christian people; and in those days they had no temptation ... they had to go to school at 7:30 in the morning, come home at 3:30 in the afternoon ... they didn't have anything to tempt them."[14] It was a simple and busy life. Lillian kept Gloria and, as she grew older, Ruth busy in the house while Jimmy performed numerous chores around the farm at his father's direction, though it should be noted that reading a book often took priority over these tasks (like the Gordys, the Carter children readily took to their mother's habit of reading at all available opportunities.) They were, insisted Lillian, just an ordinary middle-class family. But it was also a life of privileges few other children enjoyed. The young Carters were taken to see movies on weekends; Jimmy received a Shetland pony for a birthday; Earl laid out a tennis court next to the house and dammed a creek to make a pond nearby, where he built a kind of pavilion, called the Pond House, replete with pool table, jukebox, and a big room perfect for dancing, which he and Lillian often used for the parties they loved and later for high school proms.

Despite the farm's isolation, though, the children had friends. Gloria and Ruth played dolls in the yard with the daughters of their neighbors and tenants, while Jimmy bonded with a boy named A. D. Davis, one of those heart-and-soul buddies that only seem possible in boyhood. What made the Carters' situation different from that of a lot of other "ordinary" middle-class white families in the south of eighty years ago was that all these children were black. Aside from the family of Edward Watson, a foreman for the railroad, Earl, Lillian and their three children were the only white residents for miles around. When they moved to the farm, the Carters came to live less than a mile from a village named for the Sublime Order of Archery, an organization established by the African Methodist Episcopal church to assist black families in need. It was this settlement of twenty-five households which Bishop William Decker Johnson and his brother Rev. Francis Johnson had chosen in 1912 for the location of the Johnson Home Industrial College, a technical school based around a sawmill, where students could learn a trade and by selling the products they made help support the school and its programs. Nearby stood St. Mark's A.M.E. Church, a handsome steepled structure rising up from the flatness of the terrain. On Sunday mornings it vibrated as no white house of worship in Plains ever did to Bishop Johnson's sermons, which started in King James English and rose to a poetic pitch of rural dialect, echoed in the ecstatic phrases of the choir. Lillian and Earl would take the children to services there from time to time, at Bishop Johnson's invitation, where Jimmy Carter remembered "rocking back and forth in harmony with the swaying bodies of the beautifully dressed choir behind the altar."[15]

Harmony was the theme during Bishop Johnson's sermons: "the sense of being brothers and sisters in Christ," Carter recalled, "wiped away any thoughts of racial differences." In truth, though, the most glaring difference between the Carters and their neighbors was not that of skin color but of wherewithal. "We had about two hundred sixty Negroes [in the community around the farm]," Lillian told David Alsobrook in 1978, and they were almost all dirt poor.[16] As she confided to Orde Coombs two years earlier, "It shames me now to talk about it, but they made practically no money."[17] Five families lived right on the farm as tenant share croppers, the rest in Archery or the immediate environs. A share cropper "usually came with nothing," wrote Dallas Lee in *The Cotton Patch Evidence*, "and the landowner was responsible for 'furnishing' him.... A man does not gain from year to year on that kind of deal."[18] "Even honest landlords like my father, who treated tenant farmers with scrupulous fairness, found it impossible to alleviate their plight," recalled Jimmy Carter, because the dependence on the landlord for "furnishing" put his sharecropper perpetually in debt to him, effectively making him a modern day indentured servant. However, as Jimmy Carter points out, "Share croppers were superior day laborers who saved enough money to buy two mules, plow stocks, a wagon, and hand tools." One of his father's share croppers, Willis Wright, was to do very well for himself via this method, eventually buying his farm (two hundred and fifteen acres) from Earl Carter.[19] The best alternative, for laborers and for landlords, was day labor, but there was not always enough work to go around. And since the Civil War, the south had been a wasteland for cash capital and had become in many respects a barter economy for the majority of the rural population. Besides this, blacks never received as much pay per hour as whites. Even before the onset of the Great Depression, most blacks in the Deep South already lived lives perpetually on the margin of adequate housing, food and health care, oppressed by unequal wages, and by the unremitting hardship—physical and mental—of being relegated

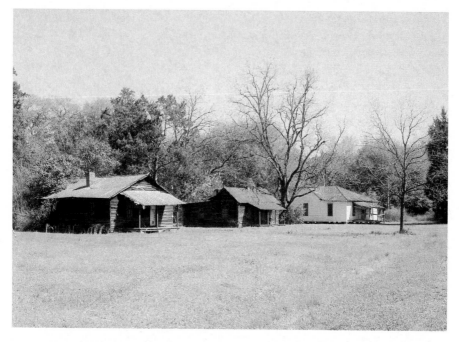

Houses at Archery, the African American settlement less than a mile from the Carter farm. Lillian spent her prime years of motherhood nursing black families around Plains, at a time when few whites played such a benign role in the lives of black people (photograph by the author).

to a world separate from and inferior to that of whites. This only worsened after the paralyzing effects of the stock market crash spread out from America's urban financial centers to the countryside.

As a boy, Carter not only played with black children, for whom Lillian breached custom by welcoming them into the house, but when his parents were away he spent days at a time with the families on his father's farms, and so saw life from their side of the Jim Crow divide. He understood how sparingly they ate, no more than twice a day, and that their food—cornmeal, fatback (the cheapest cut from a hog), molasses, sweet potatoes—was more to fill than to nourish. "The combination of constant heavy work, inadequate diet, and excessive use of tobacco," remembered Carter, "was devastating to the health of our poorer neighbors."[20] This troubled Lillian. She was a devout believer in the health-giving properties of a nutritious diet, the precepts of which she picked up from Dr. Thad Wise, who like modern physicians looked to what his patients ate when diagnosing illnesses. It wasn't expensive for poor families to grow more vegetables, but ignorance

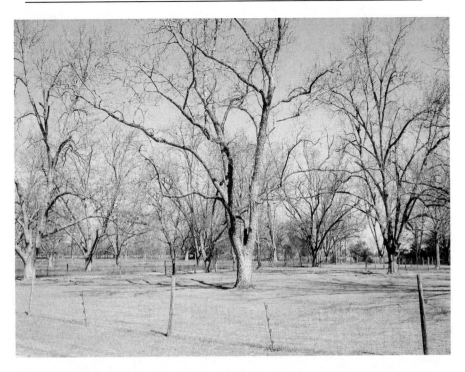

Pecan trees planted on the Carter farm by Jimmy Carter over seventy years ago. Lillian would help with the harvest, even to climbing the tallest of the trees. She hauled twenty or more sacks of nuts into Americus in a pick up truck, where she got the best price from a knowledgeable Lebanese merchant, Elias Attyah, money which equaled the fees of an entire year's nursing (photograph by the author).

or unwillingness played only a small part in the tenants' lack of kitchen gardens. Such gardens required time, energy and know-how that these families usually didn't have; they also required an encouragement they rarely received. Lillian urged the farm's tenants to grow more vegetables, and to those who couldn't she gave surplus produce from the Carter gardens, where vegetables and fruit grew in seed catalog profusion.

The six dollar fee Lillian normally charged for nursing was often beyond the means of the people she treated. As Jimmy Carter remembered, those of Lillian's patients who could do so "would usually bring her what they could afford—a young pig, some chickens, a few dozen eggs, or perhaps blackberries or chestnuts." In later years, Lillian herself was adamant about the pay issue. "I didn't do nursing for money," she insisted, and she didn't need to.[21] "In more cases than were mentioned till after his death," remembered Jimmy Carter, "Daddy provided money to Mama for buying needed medicines, and she waived payment for nursing."[22] Earl backed Lillian in another endeavor as well. "Based on a longstanding agreement between her and Daddy," wrote Jimmy Carter, "all the pecan trees on our land belonged to her." Next to the farmhouse still stand dozens of Lillian's pecan trees, some of which Jimmy Carter planted over seventy years ago. Lillian was a vigorous pecan farmer, even climbing the trees herself; she hauled twenty or more sacks of nuts into Americus in a pick up truck, where she got the best price from a knowledgeable Lebanese merchant, Elias Attyah, money which equaled the fees of an entire year's nursing. This enabled her to buy ready-made clothing for her children and swelled the family's coffers, so that even during the Depression, their financial position made it possible for the Carters to help those less fortunate in the community, as few people were then capable of doing.[23] Lillian also had Dr. Sam supporting her professionally in all her community nursing work. "He said if I would [nurse in the community], and he had somebody who couldn't pay, if I would nurse them through the worst of their illness, he would [provide medical care] for nothing," she remembered.[24] Dr. Sam would fill prescriptions for patients based on Lillian's assessment of their condition, so that in many cases she served as what we would now term a nurse-practitioner. Her gift for diagnostics, which she sometimes seemed able to practice just by looking at a patient, her ability to know who needed help most urgently, and her talent for comforting as well as curing developed and deepened on these visits to those too sick to travel and too poor to pay for it. Lillian went where Dr. Sam could not go, bringing with her the expertise gained at the Sanitarium and her inborn gift for easing pain and fear which decades later in India would calm the most distraught of her patients.

Lillian's private duty schedule at Wise Sanitarium had required twelve hour days. "After a few years of this," wrote Jimmy Carter, "as Daddy's income increased and when none of our family required her close attention, Mama decided to shift to private duty in people's homes."[25] While this allowed her schedule to be more flexible, it also meant that when Lillian was on duty she was away from home for twenty hours at a stretch. Unlike most farmwives of Webster County, she had the luxury of household help, black women who minded the children, cleaned the house and cooked. There were many days when the children didn't see their mother at all, especially when her off duty hours began well after they were in bed. One of the women who worked in the Carter house, Rachel Clark, said later that sometimes Lillian was away every day of the week. "She'd go whenever she took a notion," Clark said. "I cooked, I washed, I ironed and I fed Jimmy and the children."[26] Even so, Lillian did try to exercise a certain amount of maternal control. In the living room of the Carter farmhouse today you can see a replica of a simple wooden desk, painted black and set against a wall, which for young Jimmy, Gloria and Ruth took on a persona all its own. On days when Lillian knew she wouldn't see the children, she left detailed notes on the desk instructing them in the chores she expected them to complete in her absence. "Much later," Carter recalled, "we would tease her by claiming that we thought the desk was our mother." Even in adulthood the desk stood as a powerful maternal symbol. Ruth recalled a time when she and Jimmy discovered the desk in storage, covered with decades of dust. "Hello, Mother," Jimmy said in wry greeting.[27]

Carter has described how his mother's commitment to the community's disadvantaged included even those whom most people would have judged unworthy of it. He remembered how she once came upon a chain gang working under a blazing sun, a guard standing nearby with a buckshot-loaded shotgun. Stopping her car, Lillian asked Jimmy to take the men—and their guard—a large bucket of lemonade, with which the boy, for whom "criminals" held adventure story glamour, happily complied. As he got closer to the men he realized, as his mother already had, that there was nothing glamorous about their fate. "They resembled the older boys and young men who went to church with our families on Sundays," he wrote; as he found, in many cases poverty had driven them to the crimes that had landed them in chains alongside a country road—a lesson for Jimmy in just how lucky he was to be giving out the lemonade instead of receiving it.[28]

Lillian had similar sympathy for the homeless men who filed up and down the highway in increasing numbers as the Depression worsened, stopping at houses for food or rest, many offering to do work in exchange. Jimmy Carter said his mother found most of the men polite, even educated, and saw nothing to fear, but remembered how a neighbor disdainfully declared that she wouldn't have anything to do with them, and that she was thankful they never seemed to stop at her place anyhow. Realizing that the Carter farm was becoming something of a Mecca for these homeless wanderers, who could always be sure of something to eat and drink, Lillian asked one of the men what made her place so popular. It turned out word of Lillian's generosity had spread far. Someone had scratched graffiti on the post supporting the mailbox which alerted others that here they would receive a kindly welcome. Jimmy and his sisters ran out to see if this was true and found enigmatic marks in the wood. "Mama told us not to change them," Carter remembered, and the hungry and homeless kept on coming.[29]

This generosity and compassion opened the eyes of Lillian's elder son and his sisters early—in various forms and at varying strengths, Jimmy, Gloria and Ruth would put their mother's lessons into practice throughout their lives, because she made sure they understood why she did what she did, why it was important that everyone try to do what they could. She sat the children down and explained why she had to nurse and why her work

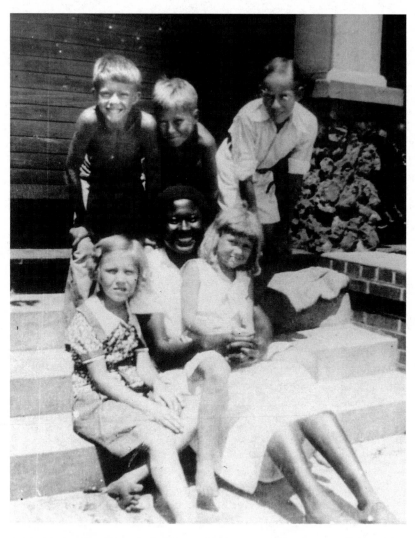

Annie Mae Hollis, nanny to the Carter children, shown here with Jimmy, Gloria, Ruth and their friends. When Earl Carter was dying in July 1953, Hollis held him till his last breath (courtesy Jimmy Carter Presidential Library).

was so important—virtually as important as they were. As she talked to them, Carter remembered, her emotions, usually held in check, got the better of her. Even then, "When she cried," as Jimmy Carter wrote in a poem, "not many tears would fall. She had never learned how."[30]

When reporters asked her about her frequent absences in Jimmy's boyhood, as if this offered a key to the President's self-reliant character or his deep faith or hinted at the feminist leanings she seemed to quixotically prefer to keep to herself, Lillian simply said, "I do believe in working women." Though she far predated the era of the latch-key child, she never found it so strange to allow her own children, when old enough, to look after themselves. For Lillian, children who had a mother constantly around were not being raised in a healthy way. "Children who cling to their mothers," she insisted, "grow up being babies."[31] This, and a disinterest in small talk that was by tradition the special territory of the town's females, kept Lillian's circle mostly restricted to her patients and her family, and led to a reputation for eccentricity she was never to shake off. She told Orde Coombs that she had never had any close friends. Part of the problem had to do with living in a tiny community where there had never been anyone like her. "Small town people can sometimes be afraid of independent minds," she said.[32] To David Alsobrook she confided that the people of Plains "looked down on me on account of my love for everybody, not only blacks, but ethnic groups of all kinds.... That's just the way Plains was."[33] Rosalynn Carter knew and admired this quality in her future mother-in-law. "She didn't care what anybody said about her," she recalled in a 2011 interview. "She just lived her life, I think kind of relished it."[34]

Whatever the good people of Plains might say, Jimmy, Gloria, Ruth and later Billy were never without a mother, or rather a series of them. "My childhood world was really shaped by black women," Jimmy Carter remembered. "I played with their children, often ate and slept in their homes, and later hunted, fished, plowed and hoed with their husbands and children."[35] Annie Mae Hollis, whose smile lit up her face, was one of these women, whose ghost stories told in the children's dark bedroom, lit only by the fire, gave Ruth goose-bumps writing of them decades later. Annie also regaled the children with less frightening stories—Aesop-like morality tales of what happened when you broke the Lord's rules (like fishing on a Sunday).[36]

One woman in particular, Rachel Clark, was at the center of Jimmy Carter's world. Rachel's husband Jack, the farm's foreman, was given by Earl the authority "as the final arbiter over which field hand would plow," recalled Carter in his memoirs, "and which mule he would harness. He ignored the grumbled complaints."[37] Jack also had the envied job of ringing

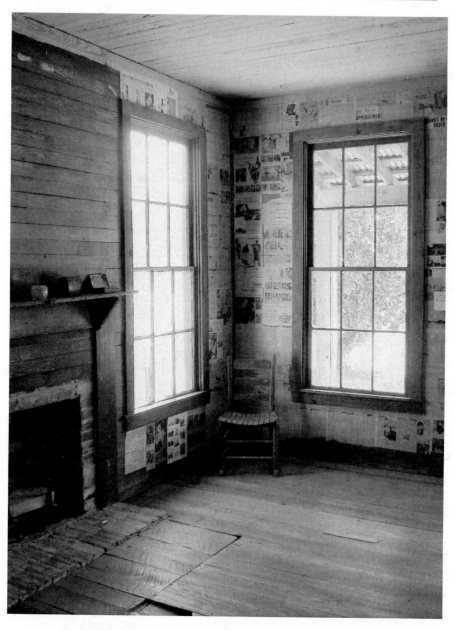

Front room of the Clark house on the Carter farm. It was Rachel, not his parents, who told young Jimmy "that God expected us to take good care of his creation.... Without seeming to preach," he recalled, "she taught me how to behave," not just toward his fellow men but toward the earth that it was everyone's privilege to inhabit (photograph by the author).

a large bell an hour before dawn to get the farm's human and animal engines started for the day's work. Jimmy remembered following him "like a puppy dog" on his busy rounds. Jack was also a mentor to the youngest Carter child, Billy, later on. "He taught Billy his first words," wrote Ruth Carter Stapleton, "and taught him not to wet his pants in a most unorthodox way." Billy had a habit of wetting himself while watching Jack build the household fires on winter mornings, prompting Jack to suggest he direct the stream toward the flaming logs and work up to aiming it properly at the toilet. "Dr. Spock may never recommend this method," noted Ruth, "but it was hard to argue with such easy success."[38] Older and more reverent, Jimmy looked up to Jack, but it was Rachel Jimmy truly loved. She always seemed to Jimmy to have the bearing of a queen—he was sure that somewhere in her family past, back before her first American ancestor had been forced in chains onto a slave ship on the African coast, there were royal forebears as dignified, wise and beautiful as she managed to be picking cotton beside him in Earl's fields. Though she helped out in the house, Rachel's proper realm was under the open skies, where she could out-pick anyone, and where her encyclopedic knowledge of wildlife and wildflowers and philosophy of what made the universe tick had room to breathe and bloom. It was Rachel, not his parents, who told young Jimmy "that God expected us to take good care of his creation.... Without seeming to preach," he recalled, "she taught me how to behave," not just toward his fellow men but toward the earth that it was everyone's privilege to inhabit.[39] As the newly elected President Carter had the privilege of telling the elderly Rachel (who, like Lillian, denied she had done anything special), "You're the cause of me being what I am."[40]

Such was the great blessing and frustrating riddle presented to Carter and his siblings from their earliest years: Bishop Johnson, his cars and his life gleaming symbols of success, couldn't risk coming to the front door of even the lowliest white household. Rachel Clark, whose precepts inspired a future president, lived in times when she had no power over her own fate, where one step beyond the lines stipulated by white people could lead her to jail or worse. It was a Gordian knot no one could ever unravel; it would have to be severed, and as Lillian and her son feared, it wouldn't be pretty.

On the night of June 22, 1938, Joe Louis fought a celebrated boxing match with Germany's Max Schmeling that on the eve of Nazi aggression stood for something more than boxing. It was a face off between a man whose "Aryan" origins symbolized all the reasons why white Supermen should rule the world (despite Schmeling's bitter disavowal of Hitler and Nazism), and a man the color of whose skin put him, in the eyes of racists, on the level of apes.

Born in Alabama to a family chased to Detroit by the Ku Klux Klan, Louis was sent to violin lessons by his ambitious mother, but boxing gloves won out; the man the press would half-sarcastically dub the "Brown Bomber" worked his way up from amateur to professional fighter by the early 1930s. Two years earlier, in 1936, the year of the Berlin Olympics when Jesse Owens took home four gold medals and Adolf Hitler swore he'd never allow another "primitive from the jungle" to compete against Germans, Louis had boxed Schmeling and lost. Schmeling had studied Louis's technique and used it to defeat him. When they met again in 1938, Louis faced not just a more than able opponent but the all too common tragedy of the American Negro: as a white European from a nation that was tipping the world toward war, Schmeling had more Americans rooting for him than did Louis, an American who happened to be black.

In the run up to the fight, Jimmy Carter remembered how most everyone at his school mirrored this ugly mix of sports fervor and racism; a Schmeling victory was highly anticipated in Plains. But hope for a Louis triumph was also high among the tenants on the Carter farm. "A delegation of our black neighbors came to ask Daddy if they could listen to the broadcast," Carter remembered.[41] As Lillian said later, "Earl invited all the Negroes to come over in the yard to hear that Joe Louis fight…. They brought their chairs, and we gave them chairs, and they sat right outside the living room window," to which Earl had pushed the battery-powered radio, speakers toward the yard.[42] They had all barely settled when the match was called: in the first round, within two minutes and forty-five seconds, Louis had knocked Schmeling unconscious, with over seventy thousand astounded spectators watching from the stands of Yankee Stadium and millions more listening in from around the world. The Carters' yard was filled with people who were all too used to being the losers in life, but who had it in them to know how to savor a win when it came. Rising quietly from their chairs, "They said, 'Thank you, Mr. Earl. Goodbye,'" Lillian recalled. Just as quietly, as Jimmy Carter observed, they all walked back through the summer night to their cabins. "They were just so thrilled to death," Lillian said, "but they didn't say a word about it until they got home." Once they got there, "we could hear them screaming and hollering," she remembered. The celebration went on for two hours.[43]

Jimmy would later write, "Daddy was tight-lipped, but all the mores of our segregated society had been honored." Not long after, though, these mores that had so little to do with morals would not be so much honored as challenged, and it would be Earl's turn to demonstrate grace under pressure.[44]

Black share cropper Willis Wright lived on land situated on another of Earl's Webster County farms. A middle-aged man of friendly, open face and shy smile, Wright managed to run a successful farm despite having no sons to help out. He did well enough to be able to hire his own hands, and enough self-assurance to decide on his own crops with little or no consultation with Earl, with whom he shared the crop of cotton and peanuts, and with whom he discussed all the day's news as an equal, albeit on the front porch. Wright was strong-looking but had a bad kidney, so when he was laid up Lillian would ride over to the farm with Earl and spend the day looking after him; she became one of his special friends, and helped in the operating room when his kidney was finally removed. Wright became a good friend of Earl's, too, who when he was out looking over the farmland would leave Jimmy with Wright.

"Along with Rachel Clark," wrote Carter in his memoirs, "he was instrumental in teaching me and helping to shape my values and opinions." In this way, Willis Wright became, like the Clarks and like Annie Mae Hollis, a member of the Carter family. But when he unexpectedly asked Earl one day if he might buy the two hundred acres he rented from him, Earl was dismayed, as Jimmy recalled. "Although Daddy had bought and sold a number of tracts of farmland around the general community," Carter explained, "this place was special." The property in question sat in the middle of the Carter patrimony, held in their hands since 1904, and was entailed to other members of the family, besides Earl's own interest in it. According to Jimmy Carter, Wright's request was "impossible to grant," not only because of the land's sentimental value to Earl but because such transactions were simply not done. Since the years following World War I, white farmers had tried to squeeze black farmers out of any land they wanted; legislation, ultimately unsuccessful, was pushed to completely outlaw purchase of farmland by blacks. Perhaps most disorienting of all, though, was that the land Willis Wright wanted to buy had been worked by the Carter family for many years, having been bought by the family after Earl's father was killed.[45]

Earl said nothing about what he intended to do. Willis's request was not one to be taken lightly, because Willis himself served as a kind of conscience for Earl. In 1940, black churches around Plains had urged their farm-laborer parishioners to make a stand for higher wages. Most laborers earned a dollar a day plowing the fields—back-breaking work at the best of times—or shaking and processing stacks of peanuts. What they wanted was an extra twenty-five cents. When the men and women on his farm accordingly didn't show up for their jobs, Earl visited each of his tenants (omitting Rachel and Jack Clark, according to Jimmy Carter), and told them to get to work as usual in the morning or face eviction. All of them complied, but clearly Earl didn't rest easy. Jimmy Carter relates that his father drove out to Willis Wright's house to ask his opinion of how he had handled the crisis. Willis, who was universally respected in the black community, was blunt; he told Earl "that the workers were loyal and had confidence in him," remembered Jimmy, "but felt that they could no longer survive without an increase in pay." Earl assured Willis he would grant the increase at the start of the New Year, adding that Willis was to let the workers know that he was not caving in to the demands voiced by their brief work stoppage. What the workers must have made of this about-face is unknown, but can certainly be imagined—these were people who lived in a yes or no world, without spin or the luxury of preserving face by saying one thing and doing another. To further underscore the effectiveness of their protest, indeed, "all the other landowners implemented the same change [as Earl]," wrote Jimmy.[46]

Around Christmas time, remembered Jimmy, "Daddy asked Mama and me to go with him to Webster County." Arriving at Wright's house, they all sat on the porch discussing the myriad of topics that interested both Willis and Earl, from crops to politics. Carter suddenly realized that his father was talking to keep from crying. "Finally, he blurted out, 'Willis, I've decided to sell you the farm.'" Lillian had had no hand in the decision, which is perhaps why, as Jimmy wrote, "Mama burst into tears of joy, and put her arms around my father." Within the year Earl, a director of the Rural Electrification Administration, ensured that Wright's house was the first in his area to be hooked up to the grid.[47]

The happy scene on Willis Wright's porch contrasts uncomfortably with another memory Jimmy Carter has from that same wartime period. When Alvan Johnson, Bishop Johnson's Harvard-educated son, came by the Carter house—entering by the front door—to thank Lillian for her help in contacting his mother in Archery while he was in Boston, Jimmy remembered his father leaving rather than remain under its roof with a black man. Lillian did not recall it happening that way; they shook hands, she said, bid each other hello, and then Earl went to the bedroom, "presumably to read the paper." Lillian saw nothing intentional or negative in this. "In those days," she explained, "there was nothing like segregation, nothing like integration, it was purely ... well, it was just nothing except the tradition of the South."[48] Years later, when Alvan Johnson was cornered by a reporter while visiting Lillian and asked about this incident, he affirmed that it had taken place, but that despite rumors to the contrary he had not sat down in the Carters' living room. In the relative safety of 1970s Georgia, Lillian almost made a joke when she said, "You can sit now." "No," said Alvan, "I'll just stand."[49]

Not long after this exchange, Lillian told David Alsobrook, "I have never had a black person come to my front door to visit me," meaning not in the carefully planned style of Bishop Johnson, who first sent his chauffeur to make an appointment with Earl (at the back door) before meeting with him in the front yard. "They respect me too much," she explained. "They'll come to my kitchen door."[50] These words may seem hard to reconcile with the Lillian Carter who so often insisted that she refused to recognize a color line. She may have been trying to explain the ingrained habit dating from slavery days that many blacks of the Deep South found difficult to drop even when it was no longer against the law, just as Alvan Johnson had declined to sit in Lillian's living room though she had invited him to do so—that this reticence to "impose" on white people was something black people considered normal for the time and place. She may have also been trying to defend the system of which Earl was a part by pointing out that the complex dance of the races, in which too much politeness or too little could make a white man the scapegoat of his fellow whites, or land a black man in jail or the grave, was one in which all took part. "Earl was of his time," she insisted to Orde Coombs. Though he was nothing like her, he had never objected to her more liberal way of living her life. If he did subscribe to the belief that black people were somehow inferior to whites, it was scarcely different from "all those people around here and all over the country who are now trying to pretend they were never prejudiced," she said. He was, as she often put it, a southern man who lived in a certain time in history in which the layout of the racial landscape was old, familiar, and apparently functional, both to whites and to blacks, neither expecting anything else. These were the black people who showed her a respect by coming to her back door, a custom she accepted without further analysis.[51]

If this was all true, though, then at what point did a segregationist who, like Earl, could support the administration of white supremacist Georgia governor Gene Talmadge somehow not also stand shoulder to shoulder with avowed racists? Lillian didn't have the necessary distance or vocabulary to describe just what Earl was. In her mind, till the end, he remained a man "of his time," a byproduct of the Old South that she believed herself foreign to but which in fact had created her as well. Not only had post-

Civil War southern women assumed the authority of matriarchs, the nurturers and law-givers of family, blood and extended. Many also became enablers whose pity for the broken survivors, and eventually for future generations of damaged men, allowed them to excuse the weaknesses, even the sins, of same, long after the Civil War lived on only in history books.

Lillian's grandson, Buddy Carter, as far removed from Earl's Old South as if born on another planet, explained this in a different way. "There are people in my life, people close to me, who have lived those attitudes and perpetuated them," he wrote in a memoir of his father Billy. "And as much as I would have liked to see them change, they never did and I loved them still. To dismiss them from my life would have been to deny the things in them that were good."[52]

"In spite of everything," Lillian insisted of Earl, "he was compassionate."[53] Perhaps her compassion was in spite of everything, too. It would be Jimmy Carter's responsibility and legacy to accept the burning challenge made by Dr. Martin Luther King, Jr., in 1963. Not only must we repent for the acts of bad people, he wrote from a Birmingham, Alabama jail, "but for the appalling silence of the good people."[54]

Lillian often deferred to Earl as the molder of their children, as if his virtues had solely gone into the creation of the four beings known as Jimmy, Gloria, Ruth and Billy. Jimmy also saw his father as captain of the domestic ship, but he knew Lillian's hand was actually on the rudder. "It was not until I was older," Jimmy remembered, "that I realized how strong-willed my mother was and how much influence she had in our family affairs."[55]

Like his father, Jimmy was hard-working, with a good head for making money and investing it and a sense of himself as curator of the family reputation and fortune that some would admire and others find overweening. Along with Earl's example, he had that of his uncle, Tom Gordy, who had joined the Navy and from exotic ports sent young Jimmy postcards that fueled his curiosity about the world outside Plains and his ultimate dream, to become chief of naval operations. "Even before I had started in the first grade of school," Jimmy wrote, "I had already decided that I wanted to go to the U.S. Naval Academy in Annapolis."[56] Like his mother a realist as well as an idealist, Jimmy also knew this was the way to obtain a university education without leaning on his father to pay for tuition. Throughout his boyhood on the farm, its billows of cotton as far from ocean waves as it was possible to be, he read all he could find on the Navy, preparing himself with the single-minded ambition that would characterize his political career. He also had his mother's clear vision where race relations were concerned, and her outspokenness when he encountered prejudice, which would set him apart in the Navy as well as from his father. After complaining to Earl on a visit home about the lack of integration, Jimmy was perhaps naïve to be taken aback when his father agreed with the separation of the races. After this near-argument, Jimmy resolved to never mention the subject again in his father's presence, a habit of holding his cards to his vest that would later give the incorrect but lasting impression that he preferred being safely mute on racism.

As ambitious as her brother, Jimmy's sister Gloria was hard-headed and independent, a bright young woman who couldn't bear to be bossed, especially by her father. She would make a first marriage to an Americus man of whom her parents didn't approve; after he entered the Air Force and took her off to live on base, Gloria's husband beat her. She left him and returned to Plains with their son William, who would grow up troubled, constantly in jail or living on the streets. Earl arranged to have the union annulled. Gloria then married Walter Guy Spann, a farmer whom Jimmy Carter described as the diametric opposite of her first husband, and with him Gloria developed a consuming interest in Harley Davidson motorcycles and the people who rode and collected them. She and Walter hosted fleets of Harleyites at their farm and became known across the country. Lillian told David Alsobrook she thought Gloria "a crazy girl, but she's wonderful, brilliant," telling a later interviewer, "They call her the motorcycle fiend."[57] Gloria and Walter rearranged their farm so they could host several cyclists of a night; there was nothing she wouldn't do for these men and women who were her friends. Gloria was so beloved by them that when she was dying in 1990, her Harley buddies descended on the farm to sit vigil, then accompanied her coffin to Lebanon Cemetery, where her gravestone reads, "She rides in Harley Heaven." Gloria, who had studied art and journalism in college, and like her siblings was a facile writer, was to play a significant role in making the public more aware of her mother's Peace Corps service by editing and publishing in 1977 the letters Lillian had sent home from India. Though different from Lillian in other respects, she strongly shared her mother's passion for social justice. "Gloria is just like me," Lillian affirmed. "We have never noticed a color line."[58]

Nicknamed Boopy-doop by her father, sweet-faced, sweet-natured Ruth was quite different from both her elder siblings, and would have a very different life from anyone in her family. Having created for herself what many would see as the perfect life when she married Dr. Robert Stapleton, a prominent North Carolina veterinarian, she bore Dr. Stapleton four children and lived on a beautiful farm. But Ruth felt a calling welling up in her that drove her back to college to study theology. Life crises thereafter led her to conclude that she had a role to play in helping others, using an evangelism not everyone agreed was orthodox. "She thinks that the church is a narrow place," explained Lillian, who agreed with her. "She is her own church, you might say."[59] Author of five books, including *The Gift of Inner Healing*, in which she described her beliefs and methods, her concept centered on a Jesus who loved regardless of presumed sins (not unlike Universalist faith), whose superimposition over or inclusion in negative memories of past transgressions could heal a person physically and spiritually (not unlike Christian Science). Lillian tried to explain her daughter's faith by saying it was "the love of God ... the love of Jesus and your love for him and not hell and damnation."[60] Ruth even managed to convert porn publisher Larry Flynt, albeit temporarily. (Flynt eventually purchased *The Plains Georgia Monitor* and in its first press run under his control he published a centerfold of Lillian in flowing robes with an Indian baby in her arms, an African Jesus spreading his arms over her head and a ghostly Mahatma Gandhi smiling over all like a Hindu Cheshire Cat—a result of, or in spite of, Ruth's efforts to "save" Flynt.) It was Ruth, always closest to her brother Jimmy, who convinced him to be "born again" in a crisis of faith Carter describes eloquently in his memoirs, a life-altering event central to his humanitarian work in and out of the White House. Ruth was credited with healing others but wasn't able to heal herself when the pancreatic cancer which had taken her father and would shorten the lives of her sister, mother and younger brother, also claimed her.

When Billy Carter came along in 1937, the Carter stage found its most theatrical and most controversial personality.

Born when Lillian was thirty-nine, Billy was apparently an accident. As Earl joked to his wife, "I know it's not mine, 'cause I know good and well we were not going to have any more children." But Earl *had* been hoping for a second son. "He said if I would have a boy he would give me $500," Lillian remembered—no small sum for the tag end of the Depression. Earl even promised her double that amount if she managed to produce twin boys, and she tried. "I would have done anything for $1,000," she joked later. She got her $500 eventually, and Earl got his boy; he was so overjoyed at the news Lillian remembered him taking the newborn infant and kissing him before he was even washed. Billy would come to adore his father, too—adore, not worship as Jimmy did.[61]

"Mama often said that Billy was the smartest of her children," Jimmy Carter wrote, "and none of us argued with her."[62] History does argue with her, with the benefit of hindsight, blaming Billy for actions that a smart man should have known better than to get involved in. And there was the press, into whose hands Billy heedlessly played, which painted a portrait of Billy Carter that could be summoned for many merely by reading his name: Billy Beer and good ole boys; public urination and oil deals with Libya; drunken capers and self-destructive adventures fueled by alcohol, which fed a larger fantasy of a crazy family of Georgia crackers running amok in the White House, with Billy as the craziest of the lot.

As Billy once quipped in the days before the 1976 election, "My mother went into the Peace Corps when she was sixty-eight. My one sister is a motorcycle freak, my other sister is a Holy Roller evangelist and my brother is running for president. I'm the only sane one in the family." This was recently put more succinctly by Andrew J. Young, the pastor, future mayor of Atlanta and Ambassador to the United Nations, long time friend of Dr. Martin Luther King, Jr., and admirer of Lillian Carter. "The Carters were a wild family," says Young. "But they were all authentic and free."[63]

Billy wasn't the only sane one in the family, but he may have been the most sensitive, and that was to be both his gift and his downfall. Compared to Jimmy's, Billy's childhood was that of the sunny little Joseph of the Old Testament, the delight of his father's older years and of his mother's middle age. When interviewed in 1980, elderly Gussie Jackson, who had worked for the Carters during both Jimmy's and Billy's widely separate childhoods, made no bones about the difference in how they were raised. "Mr. Jimmy, he always had to do," she explained. "But Billy, he just never had no business about him."[64] Lillian didn't care for criticism of any of her children but particularly not of Billy, and though she may have ignored Gussie's frank opinion she would hit back at others, fueling the fire instead of extinguishing it.

Billy was, by any standard, more than a little spoiled. Where Jimmy looked up to his father as a subaltern does a commanding officer, Billy had a casual attitude toward Earl that surprised Jimmy on many occasions. Jimmy tells of the time he was with his parents on a sultry summer day, talking in the kitchen of the red brick house they had built and moved to in Plains. Teenaged Billy sauntered in and declared he was going to take a shower before going out. "Billy," admonished Earl, "this is the third shower today, and you don't need it." Billy blithely ignored this and took his shower; then to Jimmy's astonishment, as the shiny-cheeked and slicked-haired young man passed his father, he clicked a nickel down on the table. "This," he said, "is to pay for the water." Jimmy couldn't imagine doing anything remotely like this, but Earl's tame response, and perhaps a show of humor, told him how close his brother and father were—perhaps he recognized, painfully, that they were not just father and son but friends, which he liked to think he and Earl had been. "They looked alike," Jimmy wrote, "and had many of the same mannerisms," a statement that is partly true.[65] Like Earl, Billy loved a good time and a good drink. But unlike Earl, Billy was never a man of self-discipline or moderation until the last few years of his life; he had an uncontrollable appetite for alcohol coupled with an exhibitionist's need to show off his addiction at every opportunity. Jimmy Carter might well have pointed out that Billy's pointed wisecracks were far more likely to have been inherited from his mother than his father. Lillian already had a reputation in Plains of speaking her mind which was to become an international reputation when her son became president, a habit that got more biting as she got older. Jimmy tells about the time the snooty mother of a fellow Annapolis student once came up to Lillian at a reception and said, "My dear, what a beautiful tan you have. Did you get it at the beach?" "No," Lillian responded, "I got it in the cotton patch."[66] Billy just took his mother's habit a step further, as he did everything. For a young man of Billy's complex nature—his high IQ and love of reading, his weakness for booze and attitude—Jimmy Carter must have been an impossible older brother, through no fault of his own. With thirteen years between them, Jimmy and Billy barely knew each other; the older brother became the high-achieving, stern figure that Earl had been for Jimmy, but had never been for Billy. This invisible divide widened when, in 1943, the year after the United States entered World War II and after Earl's energetic lobbying of their local congressman, Jimmy was accepted at the United States Naval Academy at Annapolis, and six year old Billy had his parents and the farm all to himself. By the time he was eight, Billy was performing chores for his father at the peanut warehouse, riding over the fields with him, spending all their available hours together. According to Ruth Carter Stapleton, this was one of the happiest periods of Billy's life. "His major unhappiness was school," she noted. "Although he was very bright, he seemed to be resisting the image of all the other Carter children."[67] His siblings' scholastic prowess and a stutter he had developed weighed heavily on Billy, and unlike his brother, he wasn't expected to live up to the same standards applied to Jimmy or his sisters. Deferential black servants and the idyll of being the beloved son of the boss contributed to an atmosphere in which Billy did pretty much what he wanted. Thus he was upset when in 1948, Earl and Lillian moved into Plains to live in a house designed to their specifications. The red brick bungalow stood within sight of the boarding house where they had first lived as a married couple. Built by local men using lumber from the Carters' lands, the house showed a featureless face to the world passing along the 280: its two peaked bays with round slotted gable vents hugged the front door, which was approached by three low brick steps. According to Gloria Carter, Earl wanted the house to be as unobtrusive and unostentatious as possible, while still filling it with all the space and conveniences he and Lillian desired. Accordingly most of the structure was at the back—only there, standing in the middle of the large garden that was tended by a black man known as Uncle Charlie, could you see that the house had two stories.[68] As if to compensate Billy for the loss of the farm, he was given that dream of every teenager, his own room (actually his own floor), which he only had to share for a year until Gloria moved out. The house had that modern gadget that had been unthinkable to the teenaged Jimmy, for whom the farm's radio had been the ultimate in technology—Earl bought a television set, the first in Plains, though it came at considerable extra cost when the men installing the antenna broke so many slate roof tiles the house had to be re-shingled.[69] Billy came to see that being in town made it easier for him to spend time with his father at the warehouse. "Billy's lifelong dream had been to work in his father's business," wrote Ruth Carter Stapleton. Earl had even told Billy that one day he would be in charge of everything. "Jimmy's chosen the navy," he told him, "and you've chosen the land."[70]

When Jimmy left Plains for the Naval Academy, Lillian and Earl were drawn not closer but literally driven apart by a shared grief. "It broke Mama's heart," she told David Alsobrook decades later, the parting still fresh in memory. When the Carters had seen Jimmy off, they were too upset to speak. "I had a car," Lillian said, "and Earl had a car.... I got in my car, and I went in one direction, and he went to a friend's house ... at another pond." Earl and his buddy proceeded to get "nearly about drunk," she recalled, and she didn't see him till nightfall. She, in a pattern that would be repeated in times of crisis, retreated to the Pond House, where she got out her rod and reel, sat on the little plank jetty, and as light drained from the sky and pond, fished and cried. She, too, returned late to the house, where Annie Mae Hollis was looking after Billy and Ruth. "It was the saddest day," she later said, "we had up until then." They were tears of pride, too, of course—that Jimmy was on his way, doing what he had always dreamed of doing. Yet that was not the end of the letting go. Lillian had another maternal rite of passage to deal with and it came in the form of a shy, pretty girl from Plains.[71]

Rosalynn Smith was well known to Lillian long before she and Jimmy became romantically involved. Her father, Willbur Edgar Smith, owned a farm and worked as a mechanic; he also drove the Plains school bus, which is how he first met Allethea Murray, known as Allie (or Miss Allie in later years). Theirs was a love match, a marriage of visible affection to their children in the way Edgar, on arriving home after work, would lift Allie into his arms and whirl her about the room—not a scene the Carter children would have very often witnessed between their parents. Like Edgar, Allie had a sweet nature; she was a soft-voiced lady, the epitome of southern womanhood as dictated by those traditions and expectations that Lillian enjoyed flouting. Though she had earned a teaching certificate, Allie seemed content to stay at home as the faithful wife, working for the comfort of her husband and children.

Rosalynn's early childhood had been a happy one, though challenging in the same respect as Jimmy's: she was her own most demanding taskmaster. However, unlike Jimmy she chafed at the limitations of Plains, finding little in it to admire. Her dreams of the wider world were fed by her parents, who urged her to go on to college after high school and make something of her life far from the village of her birth. But with her ambition went an almost pathological shyness, which she had inherited from her mother, along with Allie's quiet strength, and it was the latter quality that for the entire family would be put to the test in 1939. That summer, the children were puzzled but happy to be sent away to camp, returning to find that everything had changed: Edgar was gravely ill with leukemia. Rosalynn rose to the occasion, spending as much time with her father as she was allowed to. She read to him (detective novels were his favorite), and soothed him by brushing his hair or telling him all the latest news. She also saw a great deal of Lillian, who served as Edgar's visiting nurse and was frequently at the Bond Street house during his last weeks. Rosalynn was often in the sick room or nearby watching as Lillian "took care of [my father], gave him his shots, helped Mother turn him over in the bed." To the Smiths she was "just a great woman," recalled Rosalynn. "Jimmy's mother took care of everybody," she said, "whether they had money or not. And my father just admired her for that," even naming his youngest daughter for her.[72]

Mature for her thirteen years, Rosalynn was accordingly self-conscious about all the public focus being given to her father's illness and, by extension, her family. Such was normal and even expected in a small town like Plains, but as Rosalynn wrote in her memoirs, "There were times I resented all the attention and the people, but I couldn't let anyone see my feelings. I wanted to be by myself or just with my mother or father."[73] Rosalynn's first clue that there would be an end to it all came late one night in the last week of October 1940. Arriving at the house without explanation, she remembered, Lillian bundled her into her car and took her to the farm to sleep over with Ruth. Rosalynn's initial memory was of feeling relieved to be away from the epicenter of all the waiting and all the worry. Awakened a few hours later, she was again put into the car without explanation and driven back to Plains, where as with the return from summer camp her world had altered, this time in a far greater way: Edgar had died in the night, aged only forty-four, leaving herself and the other three children. Though he had left some money, and there was some income from the farm, Allie had to make ends meet; she eventually worked for the Plains post office, but at first she hired out as seamstress. Rosalynn helped her, and through working with her mother developed a gift for copying and adapting store-bought designs. The smartly dressed Rosalynn Smith grew into a young woman of arresting sweetness, neatness and style, but one who would always have about her the air of naiveté that would fool many people until they came to know and appreciate her.

From an early age, Rosalynn had an ability to quickly take in the facts of any problem or situation, a trait she shared with Lillian. It was also one which woke her in girlhood to the inequities of the south. The Smiths had had little daily contact with black people, because they lived in town and never had black help on the farm or in the house as the Carters did. So Rosalynn would never forget the time a black woman, Annie B. Floyd, came to her house to ask for her help with her thesis. Annie was attending a blacks-only college, an ironic consequence both of greater opportunities created by emancipation and the strict racial separation dictated by the Jim Crow laws which promoted inequality. Rosalynn found that the school wasn't just separate, it was also extremely unequal. "When I looked at her paper," she wrote, "I was amazed to find it was grammar school level." Annie turned in the paper, heavily corrected by Rosalynn, and she was proud to have it come back with a passing grade, but Rosalynn found this revelation "a shocking experience." Yet as she pointed out later, "this was the South of the forties, and challenging the status quo was inconceivable."[74]

As a friend of Ruth's, and as a girl whose father was a patient of his mother's, at first Rosalynn meant little more than that to Jimmy, whose thoughts were occupied by ships and submarines. They had known of each other for years, and she'd bought ice cream from him when he was selling cones with his cousin Hugh on the main street of Plains. It was only in 1944, when Rosalynn graduated from high school and a year after Jimmy headed for Annapolis, that she "fell in love with Jimmy's picture," which was hanging on a wall of Ruth's bedroom. "I thought he was the most hand-some young man I had ever seen," she recalled.[75] Ruth idolized Jimmy and was fascinated by Rosalynn's interest in him. She tried to set up meetings between them when Jimmy was home from the Naval Academy but fate seemed always to intervene. Only when she and Ruth were spending the day together cleaning the Pond House after a party did Rosalynn and Jimmy talk to each other. While she was sure she hadn't made much of an impres-sion, Jimmy later invited her out to a movie. "And on the way home," Ros-alynn wrote, "he kissed me."[76] So began a romance that was to heat up and cool and reheat and finally stay that way, through the bombing of Hiroshima and Nagasaki and the post-victory Christmas that followed. Jimmy gave Rosalynn a compact made of silver and engraved with the Carter family endearment: "ILYTG" ("I love you the goodest"), a saying Earl had bequeathed to his children. He then proposed to her. She, with her mind set on the college education she had promised her father she would achieve, said no; but when Jimmy asked her again a few months later, she agreed to become his wife.

When told of the engagement, Allie gladly gave her blessing after being assured that Rosalynn had thought through her decision carefully. The response from Earl and, especially, Lillian, was allegedly more dramatic and would become the subject of controversy as differing versions of the event circulated in memoirs and interviews. In her autobiography, Rosalynn wrote that Earl was clearly unhappy with Jimmy's choice. "He was ambitious for Jimmy, had great plans for him," she recalled, "and being married to an eighteen-year-old girl from Plains was not one of them."[77] Jimmy's first cousin Hugh Carter, who later became a senator and was one of Jimmy's boon companions throughout childhood, remembered a different scenario: that Lillian preferred that Jimmy make a more advantageous match from Plains, namely the daughter of Dr. Bowman Wise, a brother of Dr. Sam and Dr. Thad, and was furious with him for choosing a girl so young and so lacking in connections. In his innuendo-inflected memoir of growing up a Carter of Plains, Hugh, known to the family as "Cousin Beedie," wrote that the *National Enquirer* had misquoted him when it stated baldly that "certainly there is a feud between Miss Lillian and Rosalynn." Yet a page later he says, "Aunt Lillian hit the ceiling when Jimmy came home with his glowing account of Rosalynn and his avowed goal of marrying her. She commented with characteristic bluntness that Rosalynn was not good enough for her son and not good enough to enter the Carter family," and that Rosalynn was "from the wrong side of the tracks."[78] Rosalynn remembers the opposite. "Jimmy's mother was my only champion," she wrote in her memoirs and reiterated in 2011 at Lillian's induction into the Georgia Women of Achievement Hall of Fame. "Miss Lillian" she insisted, "was always for the underdog."[79] Rosalynn was very far from being "from the wrong side of the tracks"—the Smiths were solidly middle-class, with connections to the Wises and other prominent names in Sumter County—but perhaps it was more a case of a lack of worldly wisdom than impressive genealogy. "I've always thought that Rosalynn had a longer road to travel than the President did," says Rick Hutto, who served as White House Appointments Secretary to the Carter family. "I think the road from Plains to the White House was an easier one for the President because of his mother's family background, and because of his mother."[80]

While it's hard to believe an iconoclast like Lillian would set so much store on traditional family connections, Lillian, like many mothers, may also have felt her power as matriarch threatened by Rosalynn, the first woman to come between her and her son. But it is not difficult to understand that she would worry that Rosalynn had not developed sufficient character to withstand the demands of marriage to her son, or membership in the Carter clan.

Regardless of misgivings real or rumored, both sets of in-laws were present for the wedding on July 7, 1946, in Plains. And as Lillian would later relate to an interviewer after her son became president, she came to have a profound respect for Rosalynn. For all her quiet beauty, Rosalynn Smith Carter was that antithesis of the southern belle, a tough cookie, "just as hard as the men," Lillian noted with approval.[81] In Rosalynn, the Carter family had gained another female member who believed in equality between races, classes and genders, and with her husband would carry those beliefs into action. And in time, like Lillian, she would also become a lightning rod for controversy just by opening her mouth.

CHAPTER 4

Miss Lilly

Earl Carter had always been interested in politics, though his kind involved not statistics or the relentless self-marketing of ideas or the cut-throat strategizing that drives a wedge into the toughest piece of constituency, but in the way people effect change in the lives of others through personal contact and the exchange of goods and services. By the early 1950s, this was what Earl was known for, and he became a familiar figure both in Sumter County and in the state capital. Middle-aged and portly, he now fit the physical description of what one historian terms "the Big Daddy of Plains," and like the Tennessee Williams character Earl hated mendacity. But that didn't stop him from living a kind of double life as a benefactor who preferred to let many of his good works remain in the shadow, which would lead some people in the future to focus on his less laudatory characteristics, unaware of the others.

"He bought farms for people," Lillian told David Alsobrook, "extended credit to them."[1] "He was always doing something progressive in the community," recalled P.J. Wise. "He served on the school board for a long time, and he tried to do all he could to better schools."[2] These were separate schools for white and black children, of course. Though journalist Orde Coombs claimed to have heard negative accounts of Earl in Plains's community of color in the 1970s, possibly from those who still rankled over his handling of the work stoppage in 1940, local blacks did come forward in his favor. One such man, John Lundy, told an interviewer that when he relocated to Plains in 1950 he wouldn't have been able to start his life there without the loan Earl gave him for a car. Cars and farms he couldn't keep from being public. For other gifts, he was able to retain cover until death. In one example, through the medium of a Plains lady named Ida

Lee Timmerman, wrote Jimmy Carter, it was discovered that Earl anony-
mously paid for graduation dresses and suits for the children of families
who couldn't afford to buy them, activity that wasn't fully clear to Lillian
until after Earl died.[3]

In the way they often do, politics came to Earl, and as politics also
often do, they made him an offer he couldn't refuse. "Earl wasn't at all
political," explained Lillian years later. "He cared nothing about it." But
when his friends complained to him about a candidate who was running
for the state legislature on a platform opposing the administration of Governor Herman Talmadge, Earl went for it, especially when he was assured
that he wouldn't have to waste any time away from work stumping for
office. It's possible to imagine that Earl's Talmadge-supporting friends saw
him merely as a tool for the governor's policies, with which Earl sympathized in any case. He was happy, according to Lillian, that his nomination
was a shoe-in. "He didn't campaign at all," Lillian said, "and he won by a
big majority," as much a measure of the cronyism of rural politics as of Earl's
popularity among his peers.[4] Ruth Carter Stapleton recalled how Billy was
with his father every time he did do a little canvassing. "Billy was active in
his campaign," she wrote. "He passed out cards on the street and rode with
Daddy as he went around the district shaking hands"—the bright tow-
headed boy sitting beside his father would certainly have gained Earl the
sympathy vote.[5] After Earl was elected, Billy accompanied him to Atlanta
and served as his page in the domed Georgia State Capitol building; not
for another generation would he have such a chance to be active in the
optics of a political campaign or the life of a family politician.

Earl's legislative career was to be a brief one. Sometime in 1952, his
robust health began to fail, and it took a family member who didn't see
him every day to realize the change was serious. Ruth Carter Stapleton,
who lived out of state, noticed something was not right when the whole
family sat down to a meal in Earl's favorite restaurant. She was alarmed by
her father's appearance—he was "drawn and pale"—but what struck her
most was that when he was served a platter of fried catfish that he had once
polished off, he couldn't eat but a few mouthfuls. "I feel sick to my stomach," he complained. "I'm afraid I can't eat any more." In that moment, "I
knew something was terribly wrong with Daddy," Ruth recalled.[6]

Lillian knew, too. She took Earl for tests, and then brought him to
Emory University Hospital in Atlanta for exploratory surgery. "They told
me it was terminal," she remembered.[7] Earl had been diagnosed with cancer
of the pancreas, for which there was then, as now, no cure; unlike now,
there was no effective treatment at all. After spending several days in

Atlanta, Lillian took Earl home to the house where they had hoped to spend the rest of their lives together, and she tried to make him as comfortable as possible.

Despite the prognosis and the pain, Earl was the patient every nurse could hope for. "Even after months of lingering illness," Ruth remembered, "his spirit was so full of life, no one really believed that he wouldn't get well." Earl, who seems to have had no illusions about his survival, instructed the family that good cheer was the preferred attitude in his household. If people came calling and were depressed, and Ruth or Billy or Gloria thought it best to assume the same mood, then so be it—politeness mustn't suffer along with the sufferer. But nobody was allowed to dwell on Earl's hopeless situation. "When they leave," Earl asked, "please try to be happy. I love to hear you laugh."[8]

Joining Ruth, Gloria, Billy and Lillian, Jimmy had rushed down from Schenectady, New York, where he was deeply involved with the work of Admiral Hyman Rickover, known as the "Father of the Nuclear Navy." And with Earl's white family, members of his black family gathered beside his bed, among them Annie Mae Hollis, who had cared for the Carter children. Now living in Los Angeles where she worked for Maude and Dave Chasen, owners of the West Hollywood restaurant that fed the stars, Annie Mae had hurried back to Georgia. She was there when Earl died, on July 22, 1953. When he took his last breath, remembered Jimmy Carter, Earl lay "in the arms of Annie Mae Hollis."[9]

The shock of Earl's death—he was only 59—began to circle around the family to reach outside the walls of the room where he died, but many of the families who knew and worked for him had no telephones and would have to be told the news in person. While Gloria stayed at the house to monitor visitors and accept covered dish offerings brought to the door, Jimmy and Ruth set out together by car and on foot to alert as many of these people as they could find. Ruth recalled one especially sad encounter in a field outside Plains. She and Jimmy walked up to a black farmer named Ed, a big, burly man who was driving his tractor. Ed turned off the engine, and when he was told that Earl had died, Ruth remembered, "he shouted out in pain and fell across the steering wheel of the tractor sobbing."[10]

Jimmy had already had an inkling of his father's generosity when Earl, on his deathbed, asked him to bring his account books up from the warehouse. As Lillian recalled, "he canceled notes for people he knew would be struggling hard. He just strictly canceled the notes for farms he had bought and things like that. Mostly some of them were widows and some of them were people who had a lot of trouble."[11] As a nuclear engineer who had made the navy his life, Jimmy almost lived on a different planet from Earl and Plains, farms, peanuts and cotton. There was, too, some lingering resentment of Earl that he could never completely articulate. "I had strongly mixed feelings about [my father]," Jimmy explained: "of love, admiration, and pride, but also at least a retrospective concern about his aloofness from me.... I used to hunger for one of his all-too-rare demonstrations of affection."[12] Ruth knew that her father and Jimmy had had their disagreements. "Potent personalities," she pointed out, "usually clash if they are to maintain their individuality."[13] Yet as Jimmy watched his father casually wipe out debts to the tune of six figures, saw Ed weeping on his tractor, and listened to the stories of poor people, black and white, who but for Earl's help would not have been able to survive, "Jimmy discovered that his father had a hidden benevolence and compassion for people," Ruth observed, "that he had not seen in his youth and had omitted from his own life."[14] As Jimmy wrote, "I was both amazed and overwhelmed by the broad range of his interests, the expressed affection for my father, and numerous accounts of his previously unrevealed acts of generosity and kindness."[15] So stark was this vision of how important one life could be to the lives of many that by the time Jimmy had driven back to New York, he had made up his mind to leave the navy, return to Plains to take over his father's business and carry on his legacy of serving as benefactor to the community.

While it appeared to be unilateral, and for a time his wife thought it was, Jimmy's decision was not just about himself. Billy *was* too young to assume control of anything; and in her distraught frame of mind Lillian was unable to cope with the demands of managing her husband's affairs, which in any case had always been Earl's domain. It was a decision which almost cost Jimmy and Rosalynn their marriage. Having had a taste of life in far flung places she had only read about in books, Rosalynn couldn't imagine returning to the little town she'd thought she had washed her hands of ten years earlier. Had Rosalynn pressed Jimmy, given him an ultimatum, it's possible she could have succeeded. She fought the decision until there was nothing to do but follow this man, suddenly a stranger to her who, once so definitely going places, now wanted nothing more than to reverse course to return to the red dirt where they had both started. That she agreed to accompany him on this seemingly quixotic mission would alter the course of their lives and of history.

"My grandfather's death affected Grandmama deeply," says Kim Carter Fuller, Billy's eldest daughter. "She told me she never believed she would hurt that much again."[16] But if Lillian, married to Earl for three decades, was the one hurt almost beyond healing, Billy, though a boy of sixteen, was also deeply wounded, with consequences that he would never quite grow out of.

The day of his father's death Billy ran out of the house, sobbing. When it gradually dawned on his siblings that he had been gone for some time it was already late in the day. By the time he returned in the evening, everyone was sick with worry. "He came into the house," Ruth remembered, "calling for Mother. She was in the back sitting room where, with my sister Gloria, she had been receiving the condolences of relatives most of the day." Billy walked up to her, saying, "Mother, I've brought you a gift so you won't be so lonely now that Daddy's gone." He opened his hands to reveal a little parakeet, adding "I hope he learns to talk real soon." He had driven all over the county and beyond until, in Albany, he'd found just the right bird for Lillian.[17]

Throughout his young life, Billy had known nothing but his father's governing presence, his support in all things, his tolerance of his failings as well as his celebrations of triumphs. That was over now. So, too, was the dream Billy had nurtured since childhood, on all those rides with his father over the Carter acres, that one day he would assume control of the family businesses. For Billy, when Jimmy returned to Plains it was like a foreign invasion. As Billy told his son Buddy years later, his older brother was an almost unreal being. "My old man, in a very rare moment, told me once that Jimmy was like a character in a book," Buddy wrote. "A character who couldn't be touched; who couldn't be tarnished." At the time of Jimmy's return, "the thoughts and feelings of a teenaged boy were not the things that weighed upon him," Buddy observed. Yet his reaction to Jimmy was not just a case of adolescent rebellion. "It was fury," wrote his son. "Fury that a man he barely knew could come from far away and take from him something he thought of as his own."[18] Billy turned to the Marines for a way out of Plains, and he turned to his girlfriend Sybil Spires, whom Ruth described as "his happiest thought," for a way out of his fury. Setting him right every time he went awry, suffering his fits of jealousy, his rages that damaged walls and windows and sometimes came close to damaging their love for each other, the maternal and forgiving Sybil "became his life."[19] They were married on August 21, 1955, the day after Billy's graduation from Marines boot camp, and for the next decade he was to find plenty of reasons to stay away from Plains. Only when Jimmy, a political career swooping down to claim him, asked him to return and manage the businesses he had once thought lost to him did Billy come back, little guessing that he would have his patrimony taken from him yet again.

For more than a year after Earl's death, Lillian was consumed not so much by sadness as by anger, disbelief, frustration. "Mother had always seemed very strong and independent," wrote Ruth, "but it soon became clear that her strength had been sustained by her husband."[20] Earl had been Lillian's reason for living, Ruth realized, and nothing—friends' encouragement, getting her up and out of the house, pills to address her sleeplessness or moods—seemed to have any affect. "To us children," wrote Jimmy Carter, "it appeared our mother had two different characters: before and after her husband's death." Though Lillian was offered Earl's seat in the legislature, the daughter of Jim Jack Gordy amazed everyone by turning it down. Not that Lillian had lost all appetite for politics. "She was intensely interested in national political affairs," notes Jimmy, "and a strong supporter of Democratic candidates." Jimmy remembered his mother being glued to the television as the House Un-American Activities Committee hearings led by Senator Joseph McCarthy got under way in April 1954. "She despised McCarthy," he recalled, "and was overjoyed when the Senate subsequently censured him."[21]

Yet McCarthy's downfall provided only a brief joy—Lillian returned to her depression. Jimmy describes how his mother sought refuge of a sort in assuming the authority of matriarch so well known in southern families, trying to make herself indispensable and in so doing creating complications for everyone. "She was overly generous in trying to meet our sometimes conflicting needs," Jimmy recalled, "but she expected in return that all of us would give top priority to her proper treatment. She was quite harsh in her criticism when any of us failed to make a regular pilgrimage to pay our respects."[22] With Billy and Sybil away, and Jimmy and Rosalynn consumed with running Earl's businesses, she realized she wasn't making much of a difference to anyone's life. Lillian's efforts to recreate the role for herself that she had had years before, looking after patients on the farm, overseeing her children and husband, came to nothing because that part of her life was finished—the problem was she didn't know what was supposed to happen next.

The situation was probably hardest of all on Rosalynn. Of all the things she had feared from the beginning on returning to Plains, it was interference from her mother and her mother-in-law. Allie was one to take a hint without too much pressure, but Lillian was cut from a very different pattern. Within the family, and sometimes outside of it, she was unable to withhold opinions or observations or to fail to share them even in moments when they were best restrained. However much she may have wanted to, Rosalynn was not one to have pushed back too hard against the woman who had cared for her father, and her, in her own darkest hours, and for whom the older woman always commanded a respect even when she disagreed with her. Perhaps Rosalynn's cool poise proved even more frustrating to Lillian than an out and out shouting match.

What Lillian needed, as she eventually and so simply discovered, was what she would one day recommend to all women who found themselves in her position, widows who were bored, irritated, and frightened: she needed to go to work. Not just any work, but work that was the same as that which had given her life meaning as a young mother—the caring for others that was as natural to her as breathing. As she was later to adjure women who, as she had done, assumed that in losing their husbands they had lost their own reason for living, "Go get your job the minute your husband dies and stay busy! That is the only hope."[23]

As it happened, Lillian's hope lay in what Jimmy Carter calls one of the Alabama university system's most hell-raising fraternities. Far from scaring her off, a hundred rambunctious boys did something even she may not have guessed was possible. "They gave Mother her life back," Jimmy Carter says.[24] As for their reputation (which, as it turned out, was rather exaggerated), he added, "That suited Mama perfectly."[25]

Lillian's sister Susie, who had married into the prominent French family of Richland, had been widowed when her husband Arthur died in 1942. Susie didn't play a big role in Lillian's life, but she did serve a very important purpose for her sister: Susie was the perfect example of a widow who refused to sit down and die. Leaving her comfortable life in Richland, Susie had gone to work as housemother for Sigma Pi fraternity at Auburn University in Auburn, Alabama, just across the state line. And she enjoyed it so much— and possibly believed Lillian needed to get away from Plains—that she had her sister come up to visit her there.

Susie must have brought Lillian to a few of the fraternity's functions as co-chaperone, since Lillian was to refer to having served in this capacity. She clearly loved being on the Auburn campus and getting to know the young men of the fraternity, many of them eager but scared, and far from home for the first time. So when the position of housemother opened at Auburn's Kappa Alpha fraternity, Susie suggested she put in her name for the job.[26] In her one page application, which included a photograph, she describes herself as Mrs. Lillian G. Carter, age fifty-seven, height 5 feet 7 inches and weight 143 pounds, with no known physical defects (she did have a heart murmur).[27] "What experience have you had as social worker with young people?" she was asked. "For ten years, covering my children's ages from fourteen through eighteen, I owned lake and cabin where all High School social functions took place, and I chaperoned each function," she replied. When asked if she had any experience managing a dining room, she writes, "No," though of course she would have had plenty of that in chaperoning at the Pond House, planning parties there, and the hundred other tasks associated with being the mother of teenagers. She doesn't mention that she was a registered nurse, though her gifts in that area were to be as valuable as being able to chaperone parties. She pointed out that "I also have a good personality and get along nicely with young people."[28] Lillian was called for an interview before a panel which included Tom Burson, president of Kappa Alpha. He took to her immediately. "She was just a very class act lady," Burson recalls, "who knew how to get along with a bunch of guys and how to have fun ... a warm-hearted lady, that's for sure." Burson's impression was unanimous among the panel, and Lillian was hired.[29]

Lillian later told an interviewer that her children were "shocked" by her decision to go back to work. Jimmy, however, describes his reaction as a happy one, and he wanted to send her off in style. He bought her a four-door powder-blue Cadillac,[30] so she would have "the prettiest car" on campus, and advised her to use all her salary for the benefit of the young men. "I want you to be the Mother of all those boys," Jimmy told her, "and let them come to you as a Mother." Little was he to know then just how seriously she would assume that maternal role.[31]

Kappa Alpha fraternity resided in a columned three story red brick mansion located across from the home of the university's president.[32] The house has long since been demolished, but surviving photographs and accounts of KA brothers who lived there paint a picture of a building which, like KA itself, displayed southern glory (however exaggerated) writ large. Originally called East Alabama Male College, what became Auburn University was founded in 1856. Both the student body and the faculty had been nearly decimated by the Civil War, and antebellum ideals of the good old days, with particular reverence for General Robert E. Lee, pervaded the Kappa Alpha fraternity well into the era of the Civil Rights Act. This romanticizing of the past inspired an event called Old South Week, a spin-off of a celebration started by the Kappa Alpha order at Mercer University in Macon, Georgia, copying the colorful costumes and even more colorful historical fictions of the 1939 film *Gone With The Wind*.[33] "Kappa Alphas

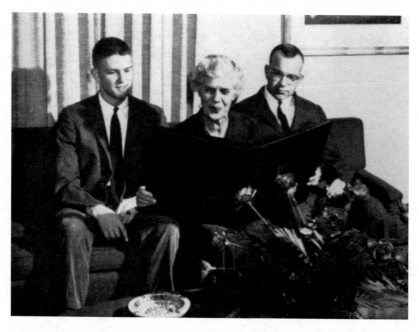

Lillian as housemother at Kappa Alpha fraternity, Auburn University. To her right is Jim Rogers; on the other side is Bill Johnson. Auburn University yearbook, 1960 (courtesy Auburn University).

began the week as Confederate soldiers at a secession ceremony," writes Anthony James, "dressed the part of rednecks at an informal sharecropper's party, and became colonels and generals at the culminating formal gala." It wasn't as if everyone saw these as something more than silly dress-up games, role-playing for a drama which had long since left the stage of history. Many KA members viewed their order as being superior to racist attitudes, and Old South Week as just a fancy-dress party, a Dixie Halloween. Yet the symbols paraded during the celebration paradoxically helped reinforce the stereotypes of a ruling white class and a class of enslaved blacks. Sometimes the masquerade went too far even for naïve youths. Five years before Lillian arrived at Auburn, *Life* had sent a photographer to the campus to capture Old South Week, and not just its carnival atmosphere was recorded on film. Alpha Tau Omega members costumed themselves as members of the Ku Klux Klan and, as Anthony James writes, "burned a cross to 'protest' secession." KA men intervened because they "wanted to be seen as civilized Southerners, not the provocateurs of racial animosity." Yet at Auburn, the celebratory parade of grey-uniformed rebels and crinolined belles that had kicked off Old South Week offered too much opportunity to fly the Confederate flag, which for the brothers of KA stood for idealist rather than racist beliefs, a sort of recidivism to the chivalry of the old south. When Lillian visited the campus again as First Mother decades later, the KA fraternity stretched a large Confederate flag (measuring 20 by 40 feet) across the columned entrance of their residence to welcome her—a touch that in the early Sixties might have been viewed with nostalgia, but one which in the Seventies, after a decade of civil rights battles and the co-opting of the flag as an emblem of white supremacists, spoke something quite different to most people. But even in the Sixties, the Confederate flag caused increasing problems as black students were admitted to Auburn and began to register complaints about them. Old South parades continue to be sponsored by other southern greeks, but Auburn University took the hint in 1992 when black students protested the parade and its lavish display of the "Southern Cross"; the next year, Auburn's parade was canceled for good.[34]

When Lillian drove up to the campus in her Cadillac in 1955, it would have been hard to realize this was part of the same country that had seen the Supreme Court rule against segregation in *Brown v. Board of Education* the previous year, but that was true both in the southern and northern halves of America. "On May 17, 1954, the most important legal social ruling in American history was announced to a nation many understood was approaching the edge of a racial abyss," writes Jerrold Packard, who as an eighteen year old Air Force recruit from the north witnessed Jim Crow for himself in Alabama. The highest court in the nation, he explains, had declared null the notion of governance by caste and color: "Americans would now have to—*at least in law*—make good on the nation's egalitarian principles."[35] Yet the difficulties inherent in implementing such a sweeping alteration of the status quo were well understood by the justices. While their ruling was a victory for Kansas student Linda Brown, it almost had to be fought child by child, man by woman for everybody else. The desegregation it promised was a long time coming—schools in Plains wouldn't be integrated until eleven years after the Supreme Court's ruling, and then only with difficulty and by no means as fairly, as was the case elsewhere in the south (where the issue remains alive to this day). Though Auburn University had been progressive enough in the 1890s to admit female students, it would not admit a black student until 1964, two years after Lillian retired, and for years black women would appear on campus only in the kitchens and as maids, black men as porters and houseboys.

Lillian must have been aware that a fraternity that worshipped an idealized south was not a place to air views on civil rights, because none of

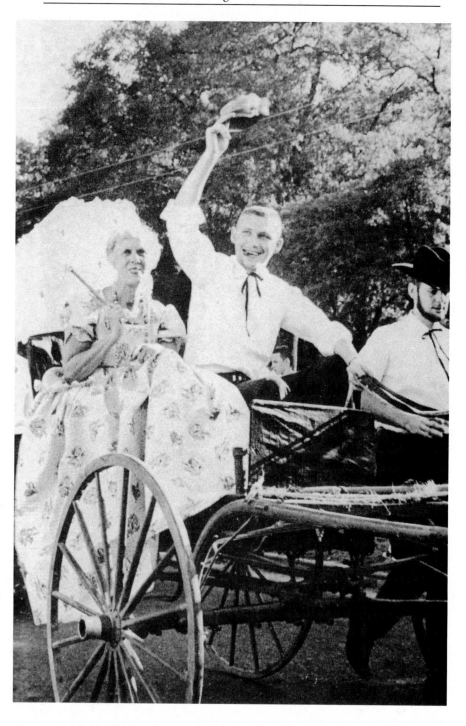

the young men she oversaw during her seven years at Auburn remembers her ever touching on the subject. Given her dislike of radical activity whether on the white or the black side of the question, she probably wouldn't have brought it up anyway. In any case, she had her hands full. On the other hand, the KA boys were hardly the hell-raisers she seems to have been told they were—most were the considerate young men their mothers had brought them up to be, which was half the battle for a new housemother. "Instead of Hell Week, with all the hazing," recalls Tom Burson, "we had Help Week, where the pledges before initiation had to spend a week contributing services to the town and to the school. That would have appealed to Miss Lilly." What really appealed to her, though, was all these boys had left homes and mothers and were trying to figure out who they were and where they were going. She was determined, as her eldest son had urged her to do, to give them a home away from home, replete with a mother loving, demanding and loyal, and to an extraordinary degree she succeeded.[36]

"She had to enjoy male company to be thrust into that kind of environment," says former KA brother Tommy Morgan. Her suite of sitting room, bedroom and bathroom was located off the main entrance hall of KA House; right outside it was a table on which stood the only telephone in the building, which would have been enough to draw a crowd to that particular location. But what attracted the boys was not the phone. Lillian was something very different from what they had known before. The previous housemother had been a quiet, highly proper, retiring lady who rarely left her room. Miss Lilly, as she was soon universally known, was no shrinking violet, and her sitting room door was usually wide open, cigarette smoke trailing from within.[37]

As Sam Ligon recalls, "One of the most significant things about the way she operated was that that sitting room had a t.v. That's where she would interact on a close basis with her favorites, so to speak."[38] Lillian had by this time become a religious fan of soap operas, to such a degree that in later years, after her son was elected president, her viewing preferences fueled a tiff between two soap queens of fictional evil, Ruth Warrick of *All My Children* and Eileen Fulton of *As the World Turns*, each of whom claimed her show was Miss Lillian's favorite.[39] Lillian was joined for TV time by several young men—more likely for televised sporting

Opposite: **Lillian as belle of the Old South ball at Auburn University. The caption reads, "A grand old gal rides elegantly into bygone days of the South." Auburn University yearbook, 1960 (courtesy Auburn University).**

events, of which Lillian was also a serious devoté—or to talk with her about the news of the world or that of the campus microcosm. The better part of the time, though, they played what the men remember as "the eternal bridge game."[40]

One of Lillian's closest friends was Tommy Morgan, and she was special to him, right from the moment he saw her. Having come from what then seemed to him far away Tampa, Florida, Morgan recalls how he walked up to the grand entrance of KA House for the first time, holding his suitcase and wondering what was to become of him, only to find on the doorstep welcoming him the image of his gracious mother, in the person of Miss Lillian. "I was one of her boys," he recalls, and one of the first things she made sure he learned was how to play bridge. Suddenly Morgan became a regular at the eternal bridge game, which often ran until the wee hours of the morning, Lillian chain-smoking unfiltered cigarettes and trying not to show too much glee when, as usual, she won.[41]

She delighted Morgan with her quirky sense of priorities. "She knew my schedule and would be waiting at the front door," he recalls. "'Come on,' she'd say, 'you've got to play bridge.' I told her I had an exam to study for. 'Well,' said Miss Lilly, 'you can put it off for a couple of hours.'"[42] Besides offering them television or cards, Lillian kept her door open to any of the young men who wanted to come talk to her about whatever was bothering them. "I had dates with the boys up until midnight," she later told an interviewer.[43] She was somebody they could trust, who seemed to understand what worked and what didn't in communicating her advice, and she knew the convoluted psyche of the adolescent male. "Some of those boys were from little towns, and were still pretty raw," says Morgan. "On party nights they would let it go! But it was interesting how she would tolerate it…. She wasn't constantly barking at somebody because they weren't doing what she thought was right. I don't ever remember her reprimanding anyone in front of others. She would take them aside and say something— she'd do it quietly."[44]

Not that Lillian was one to approve bending rules without a reason, and the men soon discovered she wasn't as indulgent as she appeared. "She had real backbone," recalls Jim Rogers. "When one of the other fraternities tried to steal our dates for the Old South Ball one year, Miss Lilly was out there like the gunslinger from the OK Corral, about to knock those guys back into Kingdom Come!"[45] (Lillian also had no patience for young women who, despite her signals to stay away from her boys, wouldn't take no for an answer. During Jimmy Carter's presidential campaign, a woman approached Lillian in a receiving line and said, "You probably don't remember me. I was at Auburn when you were a housemother there. I dated some of the boys in the fraternity." Lillian replied, "I remember you. And I remember I never did like you either.")[46]

Though on her application form she had denied having any experience running a dining room, Lillian had strict dinner time rules which nobody dared disobey (careful to set a good example, she even seems to have dropped her own beloved bad habit of reading a book over dinner). All the men dined in a room in the basement of the house, which also contained the kitchen. "She made everybody stay upstairs," recalls Tommy Morgan. "When the cooks let us know that the tables were ready for us, they'd ring some sort of bell and Lilly would be the first one down the stairs. She was escorted to her seat, and she waited till everybody got into the room, and nobody better dare take his place till she was seated. She always wanted her chair pulled out for her—for somebody to seat her properly. When she got up—usually she was one of the last ones still eating, but there'd be a dozen or so guys still seated over their dinner—whoever was still in the room rose as she did. We always did that with her, including when she first entered any room where we were at the start of each day. Everybody would stand up and say, 'Good morning, Miss Lilly.'"[47]

Lillian could be "a real pistol," as one of her boys admiringly remembers—she even began to pick up college boy slang—but she saw herself as being personally responsible for every single one of the young men in her care, and was fiercely loyal, to the point where she would even try to protect the men from their own parents. Jim Rogers, known as Jimbo, was a case in point. In his junior year at Auburn, he says, "I got this wild hair up my rear end that was I was going to run away to South America. Just drop out of school and go. I was in on a naval ROTC scholarship and that would have been a violation of that, among other things!" He was set to take off with a roommate, but when his cohort decided it was safer to stay put Jimbo found another friend to hitchhike with him. They made it as far as Corpus Christi, Texas, where Jimbo's mother, "also a real pistol" according to her son, caught up with them. "After she'd called me a jackass a few times on the phone, I came back," recalls Rogers. What struck his mother breathless, though, was that Lillian, who had known all along about the escape plot, never told Jimbo's parents. "My mother was incensed," he says, "that Miss Lilly hadn't called to tattle on us. Her loyalty was to her boys, not to their parents. And she liked to be on the side of the rebel.'"[48]

That sense of being a co-conspirator in the boys' fun led Lillian to lend out her Cadillac to those who needed it to impress a date. Tommy Morgan remembered that some of the guys abused this privilege. But at

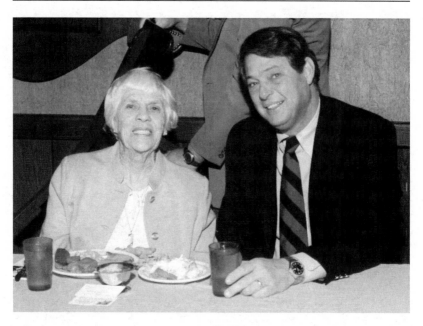

Bill Jordan and Lillian Carter, 1980. "I still think Miss Lilly would have made a better president," he declares. Lillian was perfectly serious on the topic. "I'm the next best thing," she deadpanned (courtesy William Jordan).

least nobody ever wrecked the car. Bright-faced Jim Rogers could always get Lillian to give him the keys. "I had some fun times in that Cadillac," he laughs. It was part of why Lillian was there. "I think she just loved being part of our lives," Rogers says. "I had the impression that the death of her husband was a major, difficult event for her. Perhaps her taking on the position of housemother at our fraternity was one means of helping her get beyond that in her life."[49] She went beyond the call of duty for a fraternity brother who didn't even live on campus. Bill Jordan, later mayor of Fort Payne, Alabama, had married while in college. He and wife Emma "lived in a little crummy apartment close to the fraternity house," he recalls. "Lilly came down to check on us and see what we needed for the apartment and came back the next day with several basic items to run a household."[50] As Lillian herself responded to a reporter's question about this years later, by serving as mother to this fraternal brood "I forgot about my troubles, don't you see?"[51]

The fraternity was especially grateful to Lillian for her superb judgment, not just of character but of the needs of young men away from their families at a critical period of their lives. "She was a real asset to us in rush

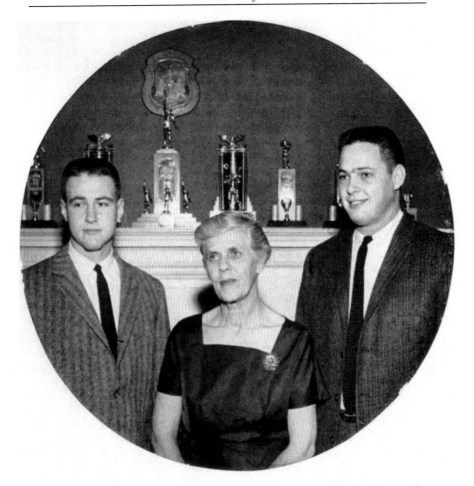

Kappa Alpha house mother Lillian Carter with two of her boys, Bill Jordan, right, and Tom Burson in 1958 (courtesy Auburn University).

week," says Tommy Morgan. "We would make sure that anybody that we were high on had a chance to visit with Miss Lilly. We would tell her that this was a man we wanted, so turn on your charm! And she would." Lillian would also give her honest opinion about potential pledges. "I've had her say to me, 'I don't think y'all want this guy....' She just recognized the traits that might not fit in from talking to a certain fellow," Morgan adds.[52] After the men were pledged, "She would always meet with them," says Sam Ligon, who first encountered her this way. "You immediately got to meet Miss Lilly. She always had a good smile—very welcoming, friendly and warm. You could see that this lady's very active, she's got opinions, and she's got this big Cadillac! And she was very protective of us." That protectiveness extended to planning the men's meals, making sure that they always had fresh vegetables and lightly but regularly supervising the excellent cooks, who were glad to accede to Lillian's suggestions.[53] She was friends with all these ladies as well as the houseboy, Joe McCurdy, who became part of her male coterie. Joe was much liked by all the men, who enjoyed "jiving" with him and would lend him money when he needed it (which may be one of the reasons some of the men approached Lillian for loans for themselves). "We tried to mentor him," says Tommy Morgan, "to keep him out of jail. Friday nights were his time to have fun and when he got in jail it was our job to call a professor of law, a Dr. Cook, and say, 'We got Joe in jail, can you help?' He'd pull strings and Joe would be let out." Joe could face this when among the men. But every time he saw Lillian after his latest escapade, he was embarrassed and contrite. "Miss Lilly would get on him a little bit about behaving," Morgan recalls. "I remember Joe saying, 'I ain't going to do that *no more*, Miss Lilly!'"[54]

"She made friends easily," Tom Burson says. "She was good at sensing who might need a little extra attention. She would seek those guys out and make sure they got it. She made friends with some of the members that were difficult to get close to—the loners, you know, that tend not to be as easy to know as some others."[55] Tommy Morgan agrees. "The guys respected her," he says, "and sought her advice. To have somebody like that was just really, really meaningful."[56] Very much a lady, Lillian could also be one of the boys, as it were, playing cards with them in a cloud of cigarette smoke and sometimes going out with her favorites to have a beer—"though what she preferred," says Bill Jordan, "was a highball in her apartment—just one."[57] On breaks, she would have KA men over to the Pond House in Plains for weekend parties. "She was a great hostess," remembers Burson. In return, she asked the men to help her when she needed it. Morgan recalls that there were times when Lillian would get overstressed and ask for leave. "She'd say, 'I need to go home,'" he remembers. "But she didn't want to make the drive to Plains by herself in that Cadillac. She'd get a couple of us and would call Billy, and he would drive halfway to where one of the fraternity brothers had agreed to take her."[58]

As the years went on, much as people in India would do when they saw her as a barefoot Peace Corps volunteer, the men marveled that Lillian was still at Auburn. A well-to-do widow with plenty of family back home, Lillian could have taken it easy. "She didn't have to work," says Morgan. "She was looking for diversion, I guess."[59] Sam Ligon speculates whether Lillian's choice to come to Auburn was based on something else other than needing to be busy—the need to take a risk. "With that in mind," he says, "I wonder if her decision to become our housemother influenced her later decision to go into the Peace Corps in India. That was taking a risk. And she certainly took one when she came to Auburn."[60]

By 1962, Lillian herself was beginning to see the handwriting on the wall. "It was just wrecking my health," she said later. "I was getting nervous over things. You can't get nervous with a crowd of boys. So I came home." She also needed the rest. "The only reason I quit," she told a reporter in 1976, "and I did quit, was I couldn't get a good night's sleep."[61] She had been the boys' "protector, confidante, loan and bail officer, and personal counselor," Jimmy Carter later explained. "For most of them, she was a more intimate and understanding friend than their parents."[62] But it was clear that being a mother to a hundred young men came at great cost, not just in financial but physical and emotional terms. "She came into the [warehouse] office one day," remembers Rosalynn Carter, "and said she had to give [the house mother's job] up. She got too close to the young men. She just felt like each one was her son."[63] When her sister retired from her housemother position, Lillian was persuaded to do the same.

Over her seven years there, Lillian had had a profound influence on the young men of Kappa Alpha. Much later, her influence moved Bill Jordan to lend a hand when Jimmy Carter announced his run for the presidency in December 1974. "Emma and I went down to Plains to visit Lilly and to tell her we would work for Jimmy in North Alabama on his campaign," he says. "I told Lilly that if Jimmy was elected, the only thing I wanted was to go to the inauguration, thinking that he had about as much a chance as I did. But sure enough, he was elected, and Lilly sent four tickets to us for all the events in Washington." His respect for Jimmy Carter is great, but Bill Jordan makes no secret of who he believes had the star power in the Carter family. "I still think Miss Lilly would have made a better president," he declares only half in jest.[64]

Lillian was perfectly serious on the topic. "I'm the next best thing," she would deadpan.[65]

CHAPTER 5

"This fool thing"

Lillian arrived back in Plains just in time to witness how segregation would meet its match a little over fifty miles away in Albany, arguably the most segregated city in Georgia.

The Albany Movement, started in 1961 by members of the Student Nonviolent Coordinating Committee and joined later by Dr. Martin Luther King, Jr., attempted to integrate the city with peaceful protest marches and boycotts of whites-only businesses. But segregationist agitators wanted nothing to do with change, or peace. Riots and jailings followed, in which protesters were treated publicly to Police Chief Laurie Pritchett's own "nonviolent" methods and privately to something quite different. Though the Movement failed to achieve its broader goal of integrating Albany, it served as an inspiration to those who participated in it and helped Dr. King tighten the message for subsequent marches in Alabama, which garnered the movement wider publicity and support and ensured its future. Years later, Lillian would say that she wished she could have marched with Dr. King in Albany, but that Jimmy had prevented her, fearing "it was too close to home" and dangerous for her. He was probably right, but that Lillian talked about it so long after shows her continued regret, along with the limitations she had to contend with.[1]

Dr. King and the Carters shared the concept of passive resistance, though from very different angles. King's was the heroic kind, shaped by his experience as a black man who had persevered in a world of white oppression and was prepared to sacrifice his life to set all oppressed people free. The Carters, on the other hand, had a code of "patrician tradition of responsibility," to use journalist Robert Scheer's words, the neutrality of which would be tested when they found their livelihood and safety threatened by the Plains branch of the White Citizens' Council. The Council existed in various sizes and strengths all across the south, with the single aim of fighting integration where cash met the till. Jimmy Carter was the only white businessman in Plains to refuse to join, and the resulting boycott hurt his family in reputation and income. But the businesses survived, and the Carters continued to stay well clear of either side of the race conflict. This, Scheer believed, "is the key to understanding Jimmy Carter.... The white elite who survived the civil-rights strife without losing their power either by overtly siding with the blacks or by taking racist stands formed the core of the New South that Carter personifies," Scheer wrote. "It is moderate, pragmatic and, above all, patrician." It's also a key to understanding Lillian.[2]

Journalist Orde Coombs arrived in Plains in 1976 expecting to unmask Lillian's liberalism as self-dramatizing or, at worst, self-serving, much as others were hoping to do where her candidate son was concerned. But he came away seeing her as a kind of real-life Eunice Habersham from William Faulkner's novel *Intruder in the Dust*, the frail but courageous white southern spinster who defends a wrongly accused black man against the prejudices of an entire county. Like Miss Habersham, Coombs wrote, Lillian had "an unflinching devotion to what is right and opposition to what is wrong" that was also "part Pollyana." He knew Lillian wouldn't condemn her husband's backward belief in the unequal Negro, but somehow that fitted into the broad pattern of her justice—indeed, Coombs felt that Lillian might be the one really just person in the Carter clan. "Although the pull of his mother's light was strong," he observed, "[Jimmy Carter] always refused to curse his father's darkness."[3]

Did Lillian refuse to curse that darkness, too, during the years of the civil rights struggle? "Miss Lillian was a quiet force," insists Lenny Jordan, son of Clarence Jordan, founder of the controversial biracial community at Koinonia Farm outside Plains, "working behind the scenes for change in the Plains community." She was, he adds, respected by both blacks and whites for her efforts, however quiet they may have seemed.[4] For all her habit of making controversial statements and taking controversial stands, Lillian was uncomfortable with rage. Yet she was fully aware that there was a generation of young black people consumed with anger, who sometimes blamed all whites as racist, and she sympathized with them. Younger blacks, she told him, were having more difficulty adjusting to a world of integration than their grandparents were. They couldn't fully know what it was like for their grandparents, who daily dealt with a level of discrimination that nobody questioned, often not even those being discriminated against, which their grandchildren would never have tolerated for an instant. When confronted with that past in the attitudes of recalcitrant whites, young people were furious, and it was right they were so, Lillian added. Yet there were ways of changing the situation that required more strategy and less anger.[5]

The battle between compassion for suffering and helplessness to end it was a daily reality for Lillian. When in India she would often lay awake at night, too upset to sleep because of someone she had seen who desperately needed help and not only wasn't getting it but didn't even know they could. There is no reason to assume she didn't feel the same nursing in the shacks of Archery. "There was a frustration I had had living in the South," Lillian said. "I hadn't been able to do anything there."[6] She couldn't bear, she said, to see a black person abused, and she yearned to be part of the fight against the perpetrators. She even saw her skin color as a liability. "I wish I were black," she once told Jimmy. Lillian explained that "I felt like I could fight my battles better if I were black.... I just figured if I were black, how I would like to get out and fight a battle that is never-ending." To many southern whites this might have seemed a shocking betrayal of the color code; to many blacks it might come off as an ironic conceit, since being black had not given them any special powers. Even as in India she solidified her bonds with Untouchable friends by performing "degrading" jobs in the presence of upper caste Indians, only after she had darkened in the Indian sun was Lillian to feel completely at one with all her patients, which was a superficial "oneness" at best.[7]

Lillian's heart was in the right place. But in 1962, her age, her family's concern for her safety, and maybe that "patrician" neutrality of the Carters, all held her back from going too far into the battle. And so, as Bruce Mazlish observed after meeting her in her home, instead of being a righteous warrior on the front lines, Lillian's position as defender of Abraham Lincoln and the dignity of black people in Plains became a sort of "status game, enduring snubs and, she remembered, holding her head a little higher and 'snubbing them back,'" and coming off as an eccentric rather than a moral exemplar. That was no good sort of life to the woman who once told an interviewer, when asked if she was a typical southern woman, "I don't think I'm typically Southern. I don't think I'm typically anything."[8]

Lillian did try to effect change in her small piece of a hugely troubled world, if not always by actions then by not holding her tongue. The assas-

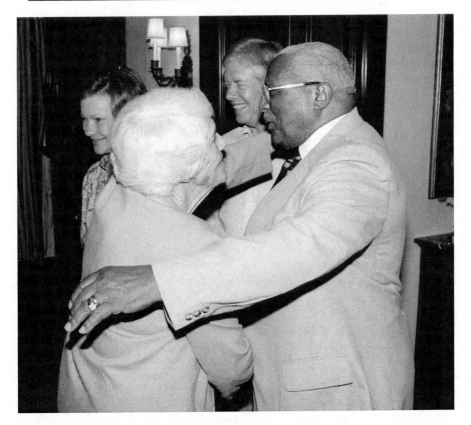

Lillian embracing the Rev. Martin Luther King, Sr., President Jimmy Carter and First Lady Rosalynn Carter standing behind them, August 1980 (courtesy Jimmy Carter Presidential Library).

sination of President Kennedy in November 1963 horrified her, but equally shocking was the jubilant reaction from some of her neighbors in Plains. Jimmy Carter recalled how his mother "publicly castigated the racial conservatives around Plains who applauded [Kennedy's] death."[9] "There is nobody in this country who loved Kennedy as much as I," Lillian later said.[10] Something in the loss of this president who had offered a new world pushed Lillian to action. In August 1964, she served as a delegate to the Democratic National Convention in Atlantic City, New Jersey, where she met Senator Robert Kennedy, another of her heroes; he later told aides he knew had a friend in the Carter family, and was to exchange correspondence with her shortly before she left for India with the Peace Corps.[11]

Following this, Lillian was asked to serve as co-chairman for the Lyndon B. Johnson campaign office in Americus, an honor that brought with it a host of concerns. "At that time," Lillian said, "people [around Plains] didn't like Johnson because he was for the blacks, and they called him a[n] N-I-G-G-E-R lover, you know." But this spurred her on. "I was delighted to do it," she told an interviewer, "took the job, and the blacks had access to the office over the hotel just like whites."[12] Jimmy Carter has noted that there were "never any serious consequences" for the beliefs held by himself or his family, but the harassment his mother experienced was real enough. Lillian's car was vandalized; even the children of people she knew screamed insults at her. "Almost every day," recalled Jimmy Carter, "her Cadillac, parked in front of Johnson's campaign headquarters in the old Windsor Hotel, would be covered with abusive graffiti, several times with the radio antenna broken off or tied in a knot."[13] "Occasionally, they would throw something at the car when I was in it," Lillian recalled.[14] Her grandsons were treated to abuse from schoolmates, coming home bloodied from schoolyard fights but never removing the Johnson decals from their school books.[15] They were brought up to be patrician too—to get back on the horse, and their grandmother, who had taught Jimmy to do the same, refused to let a little crude opposition ruin her day. "It didn't bother me," Lillian said. "Johnson won. And I won out on that one."[16]

Lyndon Johnson had basically written off the Deep South, reasoning that there was no point campaigning there from a platform that included the most far reaching civil rights legislation yet seen. But a grateful Lady Bird Johnson, Vice President Hubert Humphrey and his wife Muriel did make a point of visiting Georgia during the campaign, and Lillian met and worked with them, and she was responsible, through Muriel Humphrey, for the first known integrated reception in the history of South Georgia. As Jimmy Carter writes:

> The Humphreys arranged to go to Moultrie for a Democratic rally, and Mama and my sister Gloria were given the honor of meeting them at the airport and driving them into the South Georgia town. Senator Humphrey made the main speech, and the luncheon was planned for his wife and a large group of local women.
>
> Gloria was driving toward the hotel where the luncheon would be served when Mrs. Humphrey asked, "Are any black women invited to the event?" For a long time no one spoke, and finally my sister said, "I don't know." She knew quite well that there weren't. Muriel said, "If not, then I'm not going in." They stopped the car in front of the hotel, and Mama went inside to relay their guest's decision to the hostess. She came back in a few minutes and said, "Muriel, everything's okay." So they all went in, and, sure enough, there were several black ladies present. In fact, they were among the first to

greet the honored guest, who never knew that the hotel maids just took off their aprons for the occasion.[17]

If this kind of impromptu "integration" doesn't satisfy any part of the contemporary understanding of establishing equality, it does show Lillian's resourcefulness. And it demonstrates something else. "She had a great rapport with black people," recalled her friend Dot Godwin, "all of whom seemed to trust her."[18] Not many hotel maids, even if they feared losing their jobs, could have so quickly been talked into masquerading as guests at a segregated party just to keep a white hostess from embarrassment. But Lillian had clearly impressed the women with the importance of welcoming Mrs. Humphrey and the progressivism she represented into an establishment that had never seen a white maid scrubbing toilets. The Moultrie reception was a first for everyone concerned.

Lillian's ability to relate to the black community, and her courage as a caregiver, was demonstrated on another public occasion at this time. Around Christmas, a teenaged boy climbed the Plains water tower, which stood next to city hall, and threatened to jump to his death. Nobody could get him to come down or to explain what was wrong, and soon a crowd gathered. Dot Godwin was there and remembered that somebody said, "'Why don't we go and get Miss Lillian?'"[19]

On arriving at the water tower, Lillian ordered everyone away from the area and asked for quiet so she could communicate with the young man. "She and the boy began to shout back and forth," said Dot. "She soon found out that the boy's stepfather had been whipping him and he had decided to end his life." Yelling to the boy that she was coming up to talk to him, Lillian, then in her sixties, climbed a narrow metal ladder till she reached him some one hundred feet above. They stayed there a while, and then Lillian called down to the sheriff. She made him swear that he would prevent any more abuse, and promised the boy that she and a deputy would go with him to speak to his stepfather, who it turned out had an alcohol problem. This calmed the boy to the point where Lillian could get him to follow her down the ladder to safety. "I don't think anybody else could have done what she did," marveled Dot Godwin. "When people would mention it later, she said, 'It wasn't much higher than some of my pecan trees.'" All she did, Lillian insisted, was just ask the boy what he needed.[20]

In 1963, Lillian took a person-to-person tour of Europe and the Soviet Union—not a vacation but an educational journey into the lives, and the problems, of people and cultures far away from the American way of life. In eastern Europe, especially, Lillian saw much that haunted her. She saw almost complete lack of common staples nobody thought very much of in the United States, though to people behind the Iron Curtain they were unattainable and even unimaginable; saw the pale faces of peoples living under totalitarian regimes that stinted nothing on serving dictators' own wants but leaving theirs ignored; saw children thin and underdeveloped, starving on a diet of propaganda. Coming back to Plains, where she had a nice house, fur coat, diamond ring and Cadillac, only reminded Lillian that there was a world outside that had none of the things which she had always taken for granted, yet with the stabbing sense that her materially rich world was missing something very important, too.[21]

Perhaps this drove her out of town once again, in a search for how to be useful. Carter family friends Dot Godwin and her husband Pete had opened a nursing home in Blakely, an hour and a half drive south of Plains, and asked Lillian if she would help them get the place set up as well as assist them in hiring nurses and a manager. "My children didn't want me to do that," Lillian said later. "But it was small. It could only take in twenty-five patients." She needed to upgrade her nursing service record, writes Jimmy Carter, and she was only required to be in Blakely a week or two till the Godwins got things together. It is a measure of Lillian's desperation that she offered to do the job for nothing.[22]

Lillian's two weeks turned into nearly two years. *She* was made manager of the nursing home, "administrator as well as head nurse," she told Jimmy.[23] She purchased supplies, hired staff and got the facility certified, and was rarely seen in Plains for those eighteen months. Dot Godwin later admitted that Lillian was not the most effective manager of the budget, in one example increasing expenses by ordering that sheets on all beds at the facility were to be changed daily. As Lillian's granddaughter Kim Carter Fuller recalls, "Grandmama never wanted to end up in a home."[24] Obviously Lillian organized the facility in Blakely as she would want a nursing home to be should she ever find herself in one. If she was sometimes the despair of the bookkeeper, she was a success when it came to managing people and their needs, demonstrating the same fierce loyalty to her patients that she had shown toward the boys of Kappa Alpha. Carter writes that one of his mother's "most innovative and most controversial policies was that any person bringing a patient for admission to the nursing home had to sign an agreement for a close family member to visit at least once a week." It was a good example of Lillian's understanding of human psychology. The system was activated on only one occasion, according to Lillian, when a patient's sister let two weeks elapse without a visit. Lillian phoned the woman to tell her she was preparing to order an ambulance to bring her sister home to live with her. The woman pleaded with her not to do so and was at her sister's bedside within the hour.[25] As one year began to roll into two, Lillian realized she was getting as worn down as she had done at Auburn University. Dot Godwin told Jimmy she knew his mother was tiring of the job when she started commenting on how so many of the nursing home patients were younger than she was.[26]

So back Lillian went to the brick house on Church Street in quiet, dusty Plains. Much to her grandchildren's delight, she resumed her former life as a grandmother, a role to which she brought as many special gifts as she did to nursing. As Kim Carter Fuller recalls, "When it was raining, she would put us on the bottom part of the stairs opposite the front door, with just the screen door between us and the rain. We'd sit there and Grand-mama would describe movies, which we'd watch through the screen door. There'd be nothing there but the rain, but she'd tell us movies, and we'd have pretend popcorn. I know now she was just trying to find something entertaining for us to do, but it was magical." She taught the children board games and tried to teach them to play the piano, "but it didn't take with any of us," Fuller laughs. Lillian could be just like one of the kids, and like a child she could be happy one moment and moody the next. "We all knew our place with Grandmama," Kim adds. "She could be impatient—after a while if she was tired of you, you knew it!"[27]

The dramas Lillian was projecting against the screen door were iron-ically probably as much to keep herself occupied as her grandchildren, as was another kind of drama for which she developed a passion at this time—professional wrestling. Long before her sports interests became famous across the nation—she was a diehard Dodgers fan and eternally grateful that she had been present to witness Jackie Robinson's first game in 1947—they were infamous in her family, members of which were called on from time to time to accompany her to wrestling matches in nearby Columbus. "Some of the happiest times I had," she wrote later, "were going to the wrestling matches and eating hot dogs and having a screaming fit over the matches."[28] Lillian would sit amid the mostly male spectators in the tailored dress and beauty salon hair of a well-to-do grandmother and fiercely yell her encouragement to her favorites, whose theatrical gymnastics she refused to believe were anything less than authentic. In the uproar over a referee's call or an especially exciting match, Lillian would even run up and slap her hands on the floor of the ring. "How she hollered!" remembers Kim Carter Fuller, to the delight of both audience and performers, if not of her relatives.[29]

Aside from her forays into the Columbus wrestling scene, Lillian's was the kind of life that Miss Allie, Rosalynn's gentle mother, and many other grandmothers would have treasured: entertaining visiting grandchildren, sewing and cooking, living a defined and unpressured existence. But as Lillian told a visiting interviewer years later, "I like to have gone *crazy* sitting here."[30] To her family she said: "When Earl died, my life lost its meaning and direction. For the first time, I lost my will to live. Since that time, I've tried to make my life have some significance."[31] Now Lillian was again at a crossroads, unsure of the path of greatest usefulness or whether there even was one left for her to take. Believing she could help her mother, Ruth Carter Stapleton, then well-known in evangelism and faith healing circles, invited Lillian to accompany her to various religious gatherings. "At one particular seven-day meeting," remembered Ruth, "a woman got sick—so sick she was completely bedridden." Lillian stayed beside the woman's bed for several days to look after her. As the meeting was ending, the woman, whose name was Mary, was well enough to get up and needed to make a flight home. Lillian asked around but nobody was able to help her get Mary down to the car. "So Mother got mad," said Ruth. "She lost her temper, barged into this prayer meeting and said, 'Please excuse me for interrupting your prayers. But is there anyone in this camp who is not so religious that they will help me get this woman to the airport?'" Lillian had always been impatient with Christianity which relied too much on the unseen and not enough on action. Her kind of faith came to the fore at a subsequent prayer meeting, this one in Tennessee. The minister made an "altar call": anyone who was willing to give up everything—home, friends, family—should come up and "lay [their] life at the altar." When Lillian told Ruth, "Let's go," she thought she meant out of the meeting. But Lillian walked up to the altar by herself and, as her daughter recalled, "at 67 gave her life to Christ." If Ruth thought she had set her mother on the path to a life of religious purpose, she was to be disappointed, at least for the moment. Not long after this episode, Lillian wrote to the minister that she was uncertain about the sacrifice she had made—whether she was ready, whether it was too much. She didn't know how to give up her family, she said, or her friends or her material possessions. "My great comfort is my bed," she added.[32]

She was lying on that bed late one night in 1966 and, like many widowed women across the nation, watching t.v. in her bedroom, when a commercial break interrupted one of Jack Paar's usually censored attempts at telling an off-color joke. Before he made it to the punch line "they broke in," Lillian said, "right in the middle, and this ad said, 'Join the Peace Corps.

Age is no problem.'" (Actually "Age is no barrier.") "And I said, '*Well*.' Never thinking I would go." As she told Mike Douglas a decade later, "At that time, I thought age was a barrier to *everything*. I wasn't having any fun."[33] Even so, Lillian went to her desk right then and wrote for an application. Though in subsequent interviews she made it sound as if it had been a spur of the moment decision, she had actually thought of joining the Peace Corps during her trip to Europe in 1963. In Soviet bloc nations, she told *Stars and Stripes* magazine, "I saw something of the needs of people ... and although my tour did not take me to India I have been aware of the problems of that country."[34]

The Peace Corps had been established by Executive Order of President John F. Kennedy on March 1, 1961. Its purpose was to promote world peace and friendship "through a Peace Corps, which shall make available to interested countries and areas men and women of the United States qualified for service abroad and willing to serve, under conditions of hardship if necessary, to help the peoples of such countries and areas in meeting their needs for trained manpower," as the Order read. Giving one of his shortest speeches, at the University of Michigan in 1960, then–Senator Kennedy shared with students his dreams of what the Peace Corps could be:

> How many of you who are going to be doctors, are willing to spend your
> days in Ghana? Technicians or engineers, how many of you are willing to
> work in the Foreign Service and spend your lives traveling around the world?
> On your willingness to do that, not merely to serve one year or two years
> in the service, but on your willingness to contribute part of your life to this
> country, I think will depend the answer whether a free society can compete.
> I think it can![35]

President Kennedy's challenge to think not of what her country could do for her but what she could do for her country resonated deeply with Lillian. Unlike most of the young people who typically became Peace Corps Volunteers, and at whom its ads were aimed, Lillian didn't have her whole life ahead of her. But she found herself willing to make that contribution of part of what life she had left, not just for America but to whichever poor nation was in need of the help she was uniquely qualified to give.

By the light of day, Lillian thought she had better tell her sons about what she was planning to do. So that spring morning she went down the street to the warehouse. In a conversation that has passed into classic Miss Lillian legend, Lillian approached Jimmy and Billy and asked, "Do y'all love me?" It was her stock preamble to a request for some onerous chore that needed doing, like having the lawn mowed. Jimmy claims he said, "Mama, you know that we love you,"[36] though Lillian remembered a quick (and maybe suspicious) "Yeah." Billy was, of course, cannier and more candid than his brother. He said, looking at her with his head cocked to one side, "What in hell do you want now, Mama?" As an amused Lillian later remarked, "That's the difference in the two." So she told them: "I'm going to join the Peace Corps."[37]

When she broke the news to her daughters, she assumed Gloria would be aghast and that Ruth would cry. Gloria's only comment, she said later, was to wonder who, in her mother's absence, would go fishing with her. Ruth was more direct about her feelings. She gleefully pumped her mother for details, wanting to know where Lillian had asked to be sent. She told Ruth that she had requested Bombay (now Mumbai) in India, which fit her desired location of a "dark country and a warm climate." Ruth was delighted. "I'll come visit you next summer," she told her mother.[38] Gloria always remembered how when she saw her mother that day her eyes were sparkling, and how Lillian warned her, "If you laugh I'll never forgive you." Far from laughing, said Gloria, she wanted to weep for pride and joy at her mother's courageous if risky decision.[39]

There was, of course, no guarantee that Lillian would be sent to India should she be selected as a Peace Corps Volunteer. One of her fellow PC trainees was J. Larry Brown, who would later serve as the Peace Corps's Uganda Country Director. When he and his wife, a nurse, applied to join the Peace Corps in 1966, they had first set their sights on Africa. "Little did we know it," he says, "but the Peace Corps was looking to put in the first-ever family planning volunteers, and the site was India."[40] For others, India was a very definite goal. Another of Lillian's co-trainees, Carol Stahl, said that when she saw the three boxes on the form in which the applicant was invited to write the name of the country of her choice, she wrote "India" in every one. "It was the most exotic destination I could imagine," she explained.[41] And Gabriel and Ruth Ross, also part of Lillian's group, joined for much the same reason. They wanted to go to India because not only was it exotic but, unlike many of the countries served by the Peace Corps, it was a democracy.[42] Perhaps in her voracious reading in the years after Earl's death, Lillian had picked up his copy of Richard Halliburton's *Royal Road to Romance*, and found, as did the author, that of all the exotic places one could dream of, India was the crown jewel. It certainly would prove to be, as she told Gloria, "different from any place she had ever been."[43]

In an interview a decade later, Lillian described how her Peace Corps processing began—with her very first visit to a psychiatrist:

I went up [to Atlanta] in my brand-new white Cadillac. That's the only luxury I want—a good-looking car. And I had to go up three flights of steps; and this doctor said, "Now I'm going to talk to you for an hour and let you know why you shouldn't go. And then you have to convince me that you should." And that was a hard job. He sat across the table from me and he told me about the hardships in India (he'd been there), about the bugs and snakes, sleeping in terrible places, and the toilets. He just told me everything bad about India. And I took it all in. "I'm listening." And then when he'd finished, he said, "Now you talk to me." And I did.

He had been to the window—he saw my car. He said, "Is that your Cadillac?" And I said, "Yes it is." He didn't know who I was. Then he said, "Who are your children?" I said, "My son's Jimmy Carter. He's running for governor." And he said, "Why do you want to leave a comfortable home, and things that you are fond of, and go like that?" And I said, "I just can't tell you." And finally he said (this man was from the North, by the way; he was just down in Atlanta), "How is the integration problem down where you live?" And I began to talk. And he said, "I understand why you want to go. You'll get your acceptance in three days."[44]

Larry Brown, who remembered Lillian in training using the term "white guilt" to describe what was diagnosed in Atlanta, doubts that a psychiatrist actually came to this conclusion. "I imagine she was self-aware enough to make that self-diagnosis," he says, "and knowing her, probably *shared* it with a Peace Corps psychiatrist." But, he adds, "It would have been unfathomable that Lilly, coming from the Deep South during this era, would not have had a lot to work through."[45] Maybe that is exactly what she knew she needed to do. Far from the goldfish bowl of Plains, perhaps Lillian was able to see more clearly what it was that made her want to join the civil rights movement, to become that fearless black woman on the front lines of the fight. And perhaps she was still too embarrassed at that point to acknowledge that guilt to anyone else but an objective professional. Though she had once criticized churchwomen in Plains for planning a mission to Africa, telling them there was plenty for them to do for black people where they lived, she had had to face facts: it was far safer in the 1960s for a white southern woman to help the suffering dark-skinned people of India or Africa or whatever "dark country" needed aid, than the suffering dark-skinned people of the rural American South who were in her own backyard.

When Lillian got back from Atlanta, she didn't start preparing for what was for many Peace Corps volunteers the biggest change of their lives. Instead, she spent all her time working for Jimmy's gubernatorial campaign. "Walking the streets of small towns all over the state," Gloria remembered, "she handed out brochures to each person she encountered," saying to them with the same bright smile that would make her son famous as a presidential candidate, "I'm Lillian Carter, and I hope you'll vote for my son Jimmy." It was as if before she left the country she had to make sure she had done everything within her power to win Jimmy the votes he needed. That she had no doubt he would eventually reach the White House was clear. As she told her Indian colleagues in Mumbai, "My son is just a state senator now, but one day he's going to be president of the United States."[46]

When her plane tickets arrived in the mail, Lillian simply packed one suitcase, completed and mailed her absentee ballot, and walked out of her house. As she told Gloria, "All of you seem elated that I'm doing this fool thing!"[47] But Lillian was elated, too, because while she was scared, she already sensed that this was to be the greatest and most meaningful fool thing of her life.

By the first week of September, Lillian and the other volunteer applicants were lodged in the Shoreland Hotel, a terra cotta gargoyled establishment built in 1926 in Chicago's Hyde Park district. Though the Shoreland had hosted such personalities as Al Capone and Elvis Presley, its frayed rooms now sheltered, for $3 a day each, seventy-seven apprehensive Peace Corps trainees from all over the United States. It was a strange setting for people who had already displaced themselves from their homes around the country, some having sold cars or let go of their apartments, for this great adventure: suites either boasted over-the-top gold draperies and white brocade Louis XVI chairs, or had nothing in them at all.[48] Perhaps Lillian's was one of the latter. "The hotel isn't as swanky as the stationery," Lillian assured her family.[49]

The trainees were a mix of twenty-somethings, thirty-somethings, married and single, and a few who, like Lillian, were long retired and even elderly by a college student's standards. "Lilly was one of about twelve older Peace Corps Volunteers," remembers Larry Brown. "Most of us were 21–25 years old, so age alone made her stand out. She was also totally gray, and very 'Southern personable,' meaning greeting everyone and telling them her life story with a lot of 'y'alls' thrown in." Some were put off by this, he says, "while others found it very endearing."[50]

Lillian's first room-mate was a much younger woman whom she does not name. "I think she'd rather be with someone nearer her own age," Lillian wrote home on September 10, "so I'll try to trade her off for an older model." She succeeded in landing a powerhouse named Dorothy Bradley, one of three other women of close to the same age. Lillian and Dorothy had much besides chronology in common. Born in England, Dorothy had worked in the U.S. as a pharmacist at a time when the profession was dominated by men. Her "aha" moment came the day she, long retired, obtained her private pilot's license. "One morning when she was up flying, she decided she had to join the Peace Corps," recalls Carol Stahl. Dorothy and Lillian befriended another older trainee, retired nurse Mabel Yewell who, despite her prim and proper exterior had courted controversy working with some of the early pioneers of birth control and family planning. And unlike Lillian, Mabel had actually served as a nurse during World War I. Eventually Dorothy and Mabel moved in together; later, in India, Mabel and Lillian would be thrown together again, close proximity exaggerating the qualities they *didn't* share. "We get along fine," Lillian would write of Mabel, "but are as far apart emotionally as a Maddox and Kennedy are politically!" They were far apart in another way, too: Mabel Yewell had no intention of doing anything she did not feel like doing, while Lillian would make herself ill trying to do more than she needed to, each for reasons integral to their personalities and backgrounds.[51]

The trainees endured a schedule daunting even for young people—Lillian certainly considered her first week of language training the most difficult task she had ever had to accomplish. "We sat on floors six hours a day, six days a week," says Larry Brown, "learning language, without books, eight to ten of us with one Indian teacher."[52] They were taught Marathi, the official language of Maharashtra state in west-central India. Carol Stahl remembers how their cadre was so successful at learning the language the Peace Corps found it had a surplus of Marathi speakers on its hands. Though they were all meant to be in rural areas of Maharashtra, "many of us were scattered around," says Stahl, often in places like Mumbai, where Hindi would have been the more practical language to speak—in fact Stahl had to keep a Hindi teacher on full-time hire during her two years there. (Lillian was to study Hindi, too.)[53] Evangeline (Van) Shuler was one of Lillian's near contemporaries in the cadre of older trainees. Living to 108, Van was just into her 60s when she and her husband signed on with the Peace Corps. She and Lillian didn't have much in common besides age and an interest in helping the disadvantaged. Van remembered that she and her husband were in Lillian's group with two other people for language training, and her recollections of what it was like to learn with students who could have been their children or grandchildren likely echoes Lillian's own experience. "In the first session with the younger volunteers," Van said, "we got along just fine—we were okay. But by the second or third session, we realized these kids were just going way ahead of us! I'd always been pretty smart," she added, "and thought that by the second or third time I'd get it, but the younger people were catching the language much better than we did ... we older volunteers were all having difficulties."[54] "Neither Lilly nor most of the older ones mastered Marathi very well," recalls Larry Brown, who became fluent. "Lilly usually covered it over with a 'Namasté, y'all,' to make everyone laugh."[55]

Lillian did make excellent progress in the family planning aspect of training. Carol Stahl points out that while Jimmy Carter writes in *A Remarkable Mother* that Lillian didn't know till she got to India that she would be working in family planning, this is not in fact the truth: family planning *was* the focus of the entire exercise in Chicago, from day one. Stahl writes that close to half their training time was under the management of Chicago Planned Parenthood. "CPP taught us anatomy, reproductive physiology, contraception technology, family planning teaching methods, hands on development of visual teaching aids, and how to talk to strangers about sensitive subjects," she remembers.[56] For Lillian, everything about these classes touched on her experience as a registered nurse. "My medical knowledge is returning," she wrote home, "and I'm getting used to being taught the facts of life by a young black man. Lord, folks in Plains would have a fit!" She noted that Marathi dialogues came much easier to her when the focus was on family planning because the phrases were "sorta spicy," she confessed, "and we can hardly wait to get to the next one!"[57] In addition to all this, the trainees spent hours handing out family planning information on the streets of Chicago, often on bicycles which not everyone took to (we don't know Lillian's opinion of them), a method ideal for teaching them how to walk the talk by dealing with the public and all its varied responses to this controversial topic. As one of the older volunteers recalled, they had to take twenty-six page questionnaires door to door in "Negro neighborhoods." Most of the time the housewife or husband or both would freely answer the questions, including some of the more personal ones, yet there were times when the questions went too far and volunteers were politely but firmly asked to leave.[58]

Jimmy's run for governor of Georgia had steadily heated up in Lillian's absence; the outcome of the election preyed on Lillian's mind almost to the exclusion of anything else, which would not have helped her concentrate on Marathi. She spoke at length to the others about her fears as well as her confidence that Jimmy would become governor of Georgia, and may have talked about it too much, as she only succeeded in raising everyone's skepticism.[59]

By the end of her first week in Chicago, the news wasn't good. Jimmy had lost (or, at that point, seemed to have lost, pending a recount) to Lester Maddox, a former Atlanta restaurateur who had threatened to raise an axe handle against any black person who tried to dine at his establishment. The final decision on the election results would rest with the Georgia State Legislature, and only after Lillian had been in India for two months would she hear that lawmakers had named Maddox governor. "I decided I had to quit worrying," Lillian wrote in a letter, "and just be proud that he ran such a wonderful race.... I must not worry about anything else." Yet a month later, she played hooky from a family planning lecture to sit in the hotel lobby, where with delight she watched senators in town for the Illinois Democratic Convention, passing to and fro. She was also scanning the newspapers for political news from Georgia and was furious to find a two pager in the Chicago *Sun-Times* featuring George Wallace and Maddox, southern politicians who were the antithesis of everything Lillian believed in. "I am absolutely sick of Georgia politics," she fumed, "but I want to hear EVERYTHING that happens." There soon wouldn't be time or energy even for her appetite for politics, though Lillian would find a use for another kind of politicking.[60]

As the only southerner among the Yankees, Lillian was to find out the hard way just what discrimination could feel like.

She wanted everyone to like her, but this didn't always achieve the desired result—in fact, the Peace Corps psychiatrist she talked to in Chicago cautioned her that some of the others felt she was "too friendly."[61] That was the initial impression of a young couple named Gabe and Ruth Ross. Both had grown up in New York City, and had never known any southerners except through news reports of desegregation battles or when they had joined in protests against segregationist Mississippi governor Ross Barnett on his visit to the city. "We had this New Yorker's view of the world," says Gabe, "where everything besides New York and big cosmopolitan cities seemed very distant." Their first impression of Lillian was that she was "bright and gracious and friendly," but her Georgia accent and her overt friendliness made them wary of her, as did her habit of telling all about her life, including what she confided to them about Earl. "She told us her husband had pretty much fit that Southern stereotype," says Ruth.[62] It was as if Lillian was already so apprehensive of being judged by Northern standards she chose to distance herself from the stereotype by contrasting her broad beliefs with the narrower ones of her deceased husband. Yet her garrulousness only reinforced that stereotype.

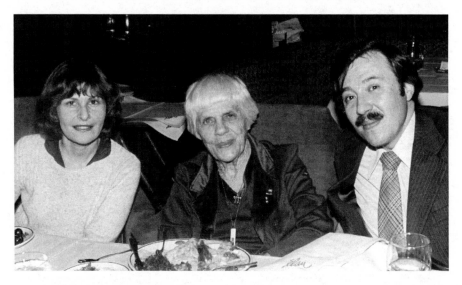

Lillian with fellow Returned Peace Corps volunteers, Gabe and Ruth Ross. In India, Lillian sent them books and reassuring notes, and later, as First Mother, gave them free rein of the White House's private quarters (courtesy Gabe and Ruth Ross).

Gabe's and Ruth's attitude toward Lillian was changed through the Peace Corps's application of Indian political structure—the *panchayat raj*, which in fact was a descendant of British administrative systems—to the way the trainees related to each other, in groups and as individuals. Gabe was elected by the trainees' *panchayat* as *sarpanch* or head of their "village government." He was told that one of his jobs was to make certain the volunteers understood the process called "deselection." "They said they were pleased that so many people wanted to go overseas," recalled Gabe, "but that some people are deselected for various reasons that the Peace Corps considered important, in terms of services in the country the volunteers were going to." What was worse, all the volunteers had to evaluate each other's suitability, with votes against an individual leading to review for suitability by the Peace Corps and, possibly, that individual being sent home. "This was the Sixties," says Gabe, "a time of activism, and my first response was to say, 'No, we don't do that, we don't select or deselect each other.' But the Peace Corps folks had been through this all before. They told me to tell the volunteers what they'd said and to get back to them with their answer." The volunteers, including Lillian, were unanimous in their refusal to participate in the process Gabe described for them. But when he reported this to Peace Corps staff, there was no sympathy. "They told me that that was fine," Gabe recalls. "I could tell the volunteers that anyone who didn't want to do this could opt out. However, anyone who didn't fill out the form couldn't go overseas. 'It's that simple,' they said. That was very upsetting, because we all wanted to go overseas." The volunteers concluded that they either had to fill out the form and participate in the process, or they wouldn't be going to India.[63]

That night, Gabe and Ruth were in their room when someone knocked. "I opened the door and there's Lilly," Gabe remembers. "She said she wanted to talk to me. She looked very unhappy—she might even have been tearful." Lillian told Gabe and Ruth that she now understood the process of selection for the Peace Corps. "She was convinced that the prospective volunteers were not going to select her to go overseas," says Gabe. "The reason she gave was that she was so much older than everybody else, she had an accent and she was from the south"—all the reasons that had caused Gabe and Ruth to avoid her in training sessions. "You folks may think that I wouldn't make a good volunteer," Lillian told them, "but I'm just as motivated as everybody else is, and I really want to go. I'm very unhappy." She and the others had already seen how one of their group, a man Lillian calls Smiley, couldn't take the pressure and had deselected himself, "and we all felt just like he'd died!"[64] But Lillian was not so upset that she hadn't worked out a strategy. As Gabe recalls, "She told us, 'You seem to know many of these folks, and they elected you. I would appreciate having a chance to spend as much of my free time with you as I can, to sit with you for meals and such. In the process I'll get to know these other folks. If they get to know me, I think they'll realize that I'm a good candidate to go overseas.'"[65]

Jim Jack Gordy's daughter was nothing if not a master of political chess. "One of the reasons I think Lilly sought out Gabe and Ruth was because she was a very savvy person regarding political orientation," says Carol Stahl, "and the art of making friends in case you needed them." Mabel and Carol were in the same language training group, and Carol wondered if Mabel was having similar fears about deselection. They were all about to go through the last test of their Marathi skills, Carol recalls, and she marveled at how serene the older woman was next to the young trainees who were sitting around wringing their hands. "I said to Mabel, 'Are you really good at this language?,'" recalls Carol. "She kind of laughed at me—she was no sweet old lady but she was a very nice person. She said, 'They're going to take me. They need older people in the Peace Corps, for their image. I do my best but I'm not worried about this.' This made me a bit skeptical of Lilly, who was more flamboyant about her fears."[66]

The Rosses also saw Lillian as flamboyant, but they knew, from spending time with her, how seriously she took the training, how important it was for her to be ready for India. "We learned later that she sat with people and said, 'Practice language with me,'" remembers Ruth. "She had a thirst for learning and she was trying to make friends and ensure she could go overseas." In a pattern that was to be repeated in India, Lillian also didn't quite follow the Peace Corps's rules for filling out the evaluation form. As she told her family, "I just wrote in the space, 'I think everyone is trying, and I believe each one has something to offer.'"[67] That Lillian's willpower was at least as strong as her fear is evident in a letter she wrote home in early October. "I've found you have to be perfect to BE in the Peace Corps," she told her family. "I asked one of the teachers about it, and he said, 'We hardly ever de-select anyone. We just make it so tough they de-select themselves.' That I damn well know! I'M STICKING!"[68]

The one part she could never feel comfortable with was the psychological oversight. She lived with the constant apprehension that something she confided or accidentally revealed might lead to deselection. Full of the confidence of youth, Carol Stahl claims she wasn't bothered by the psychiatrists who spent so much time with her and the other trainees, and believes too much was made of this by Lillian later on. "I think she was just not accustomed to that much inspection of her motives," she says.[69] (What none of the trainees knew at the time, but which Lillian became apprised of years later, was that the FBI *had* done studies on each person—so the scrutiny went much deeper than anybody knew.)[70]

Larry Brown saw the scrutiny differently. "The psychiatric stuff was both over the top and downright silly," he says. "Five to six psychiatrists who had never been to India and not knowing what type of personality worked best there, observing our every move."[71] Gabe Ross, who became a psychologist, looks back on the surveillance with doubts. "The University of Chicago was one of the best graduate schools of psychology," he says, "but I still wondered, even later, when I had the same training, how appropriate some of the probing was." Lillian was probably worrying far more than she needed to. The psychiatrist who watched and talked to her seems to have come to the conclusion that to tamper too much with her authenticity would be catastrophic. Though he, as before, still judged her "too friendly," he told her at length, "Don't try to change your personality, Mrs. Carter, you'd be a mess!"[72]

Lillian found her friends mostly among the younger trainees and formed attachments which were to last far longer than any of them realized. "Some people here I love," she wrote, "some I like—some I like and love— some I love and don't like—and some I purely do NOT like." Besides Larry,

Gabe, and Ruth, she befriended Holt (later Jules) Quinlan, a bearded graduate of Harvard Divinity School whom she described to her family as looking "just like Jesus." (The Rosses describe him as "a spiritual person of a
secular persuasion," characteristics with which Lillian could identify.)[73]
Holt clearly came under the like *and* love category. Lillian had discussions
with him about religion and the Bible; when he asked her what her favorite
chapter was, she told him it was the Epistle to Philemon, the imprisoned
Apostle Paul's letter to his friend about Philemon's slave Onesimus, who
had run away and stolen his master's goods. "We read it together," Lillian
wrote, "and had a little prayer. It was a wonderful time—one I'll always
remember." About all the trainees, she told her family, "These are some of
the loveliest people I have ever known"—not just people she had suffered
with through Marathi tests and deselections and bike rides through
whizzing Chicago traffic, but people she could call her friends.[74]

Van Shuler's teacher told her in late October that "we Peace Corps
trainees [are] at battle Fatigue stage now." It was an assessment with which
Lillian would have agreed. But by mid–November, the exams were done.
Lillian's consisted of having to stand in front of her Indian teacher, a small,
attractive lady to whom Lillian had taken an immediate liking (and had
possibly charmed herself), and in Marathi count to fifty, and speak a set
phrase introducing herself and explaining that she had come to India to
teach family planning. Her teacher laughed. "My God, Lilly," she exclaimed,
"I didn't understand a word you said." But she passed her and, as Lillian
wrote home, "I felt so *good*."[75] On November 18th Lillian wrote joyfully
that "I feel wonderful, excited, and I love everybody," though in a letter she
wrote on the last day of the month, less than two weeks till she got on the
plane for India, she confided, "I'm a little scared. All this India stuff may
SOUND romantic, but deep within me, I know there's another side to it....
That world beyond is just a great big IF and WHEN.... But, I know that
when I get somewhere, I'll be O.K."[76]

Lillian did have one final fright at Kennedy Airport. She was met by
reporters and television crew, and the hustle and bustle so confused her
she couldn't find the other volunteers she was traveling with. She then
heard her name being paged throughout the terminal. "The only thing I
could think of," she said later, "was, 'My God, I've been de-selected!'" But
it was just a press photographer eager to take a few shots before she got on
the plane. By this time one of the volunteers had caught up with her and
was marveling at all the attention. "Lilly," he said, "that IS fame!"[77]

PART II.
THE EYE OF GOD

U.S. relations with India will either be very good, or they will be destroyed by the time Mama gets back.

—Jimmy Carter

CHAPTER 6

Mother India

Like one of her fellow Peace Corps Volunteers, Lillian probably awakened her first morning in New Delhi to the pungent smell of burning cow paddies—definitely not a bovine odor she would have encountered on the farm at Archery. From her hotel window, she could have looked out, as Volunteer Fran Kennedy did, to see that "colorful saris already washed dried on the ground, over railings, or any place they could fit," or hear the fruit wallahs calling their produce through streets crowded with early rickshaws while a snake charmer piped enchantments outside the door of the hotel. "My heavens, in Georgia we run from snakes," Lillian said later.[1]

From her arrival in the Indian capital, Lillian was not thrown heedless into an alien culture: not for Senator Carter's mother the slums and squalor she had read about back home. Lillian was guided by reporters through gardens filled with emerald parrots, bused out to Agra to scoot in cloth booties through the Taj Mahal, and invited to the American Embassy, where Ambassador Chester Bowles gave a speech to the Volunteers which Lillian claimed put her into a sound sleep. "I guess we're being indoctrinated," she quipped afterward in a letter to her family—coming from a woman who had been anti-indoctrination all her life, this comment was probably only half in jest. In Chicago, Lillian had already had her misgivings about what the Peace Corps expected her to do in India. Now that she was there, she sensed that the India she had come to find—in which she hoped her skills would make a difference—was very far from the brightly lit and comfortable rooms of the embassy that welcomed her. She knew that beyond the gates of her hotel, in the narrow alleys outside the tourist districts, were men, women and children who had absolutely nothing.

When she looked into the faces of waiters carrying platters of food to people who had never had to do without it for a day, she could see hunger in their eyes. "I'm beginning to realize," Lillian wrote to her family, "how different it is here."[2]

From New Delhi, Lillian boarded a train with Mabel Yewell, who was assigned to be her room-mate. They headed south on a thirteen hour trip to Mumbai, then (and until 1996) called Bombay, traveling a total of nearly nine hundred miles. Besides the overcrowded conditions, the women endured a dust bath throughout much of the journey. "It finally got so thick," Lillian complained in a letter, "it just sifted through and went out the other side of the train." Mabel doesn't seem to have minded. As she told a reporter before leaving the U.S., when asked if she wouldn't mind living as the Indians did, "You figure when I was a child they had no indoor toilets, and I slept in a room with no central heating"—she would have no problem with Spartan conditions, she assured the journalist. This hardiness had endeared Mabel to Carol Stahl in Chicago but did not impress Lillian, whose dramatic reactions required a response Mabel was constitutionally unable to give. Perhaps this is why she added to her letter, "[Mabel and I] will soon hate each other, I'm sure."[3]

They arrived in Mumbai less than a week before Christmas, and even in temperatures which to a southerner like Lillian were more appropriate for summer there were Christmas trees, Santa Clauses, and decorations put up by the Mumbai Christian community. Such was the diversity of this city, which had been a Portuguese and then a British colony for several hundred years, filled with many cultures, faiths and sects. To this mix was added great wealth developed from international trade, and alongside the wealth, grinding poverty. Carol Stahl and Jules Quinlan, among the few Volunteers assigned to Mumbai proper, recalled the shock of the "hutments" or flimsy shelters made from cardboard boxes in which whole families lived on the streets. "The sidewalks were the only home for hundreds of thousands of people in Mumbai," recalled Quinlan.[4] This poverty was, of course, part of the vicious circle of a society that created more children than it could feed, and the hutments a microcosm of the vaster situation throughout India. The Volunteers of India 39, most of whom were assigned to villages scattered around Maharashtra state, were walking straight into a face off between Prime Minister Indira Gandhi and an exploding birthrate that nothing seemed able to control. Maharashtra had been the first Indian state to implement a family planning program (in 1956), followed by other states. But as Dr. S.N. Agarwala, Princeton-educated head of the Demographic Research Centre in New Delhi, wrote in 1966, family planning in India "has so far met with only marginal success." India's population that year stood at 494 million persons. Dr. Agarwala found that only 2.4 percent of reproductive couples, most of whom were in the 20–29 age bracket, were actually using contraceptives. If India intended to meet the goals it had set for itself for the next decade, he wrote, "this can be achieved only if the States increase their efforts by two to three thousand percent"—obviously a far from realistic benchmark.[5]

When Hindu writer Ved Mehta visited a family planning center in New Delhi around this time, he found "a one-room shack set in one of the countless slums of the city that are washed by open drains." The doctor in charge told Mehta that "fifteen years, twenty-six billion rupees, and the efforts of three Five-Year Plans have all achieved nothing." There were not enough doctors to implement mass sterilization, she went on, and men in the villages "associate sterilization with castration, so most of them won't hear of the operation." Another problem was the lack of women doctors. No Indian woman would ever submit to a gynecological examination carried out by a male physician. One of the problems the doctor cited, confirmation of which can be found in S.N. Agarwala's report, is that IUCDs—considered a reliable form of contraception in a society where men rarely took the initiative—tended to cause bleeding, which was especially endemic in women who were anemic and undernourished (which constituted most of the reproductive mothers of India). Another doctor advised giving these women iron supplements. "Of course," Mehta points out, "the problem of paying for these medicines remains."[6] Though in 1966 she contented herself with the Peace Corps' comparatively benign, and free, assistance in bringing family planning concepts and techniques to Maharashtra state, it would take another decade before Indira Gandhi imposed forced sterilization (carried out by her son Sanjay) on her country's poor during India's 1975–1977 Emergency, with results still controversial to this day.

Months before Lillian's arrival, Mrs. Gandhi had more to worry about than the birthrate. "India in January 1966 was in worse shape than it had ever been under either Nehru or Shastri," writes Mrs. Gandhi's biographer Kathleen Frank. Drought, famine, riots, a flagging economy, threatened secession, and difficult relations with the United States after the Americans provided arms to Pakistan were all on Mrs. Gandhi's table.[7] And attitudes to India's first female prime minister—called by one detractor a "dumb doll"—and Mrs. Gandhi's stumbles early in her premiership seem to have filtered down to Lillian, who was to view her with a jaundiced eye well past her period of service.

⊰◈⊱

Lillian and Mabel were assigned to Vikhroli, a unique place that was a kind of compromise between city and countryside. Only fifteen miles from the gridlocked traffic of downtown Mumbai, Vikhroli was the manufacturing base of the Godrej Group, more of a company town than the village Lillian would often refer to. Founded over a half century earlier by Ardeshir and Pirojsha Godrej, the family conglomerate had had its start in the manufacturing of safes and heavy equipment, eventually encompassing everything from word processors to soap to refrigerators to rocket launchers. Rich even by Mumbai's gilded standards, the Godrej family used their wealth to create an infrastructure in Vikhroli to take care of the needs of their many employees, which included their widows and children. Lillian and Mabel were provided an apartment in the Vikhroli Hillside Colony, a mile's walk by dirt road from where they would work. The apartment (address 13/6) had two bedrooms, a living room, a kitchen (with refrigerator and stove, though there was not a Western-style sink), a bathroom and a balcony looking out at the nearby hills, which at night glowed with fires lit by the very poor dwelling in grass and mud huts. Lillian acknowledged that "we live in luxury compared even to some of the other PCVs," and indeed the apartment building was only for the use of upper level Godrej staff.[8] Carol Stahl believes Lillian was not sent there by chance. "We always assumed that her son being who he was, the Peace Corps was more careful with her," says Stahl of Lillian. "She had more amenities in Vikhroli than we did with the whole of Mumbai at our feet." The more youthful volunteers didn't begrudge her this, she adds. "We were young and tough and thought we could handle anything."[9]

Among Vikhroli's landscaped gardens and avenues of *ashoka* trees were factories for the various industries, houses for the men and women who spent most of their day working in them, a canteen, a school for children, and a single story stucco welfare station called *Pragati Kendra* (Progress Center). Kendra, as Lillian called it, was run by a warm-hearted but, according to Lillian, sometimes imperious woman named Aloo K. Mowdawala, under whose supervision widows and children of Godrej employees received employment and care. It was at Kendra that Lillian was to begin her family planning work by looking after the records of the well-baby clinic, school health, family planning and other family health programs. She was also tasked with visiting families to explain to them what family planning was all about, visits she had to make with a native speaker in tow as her Marathi consisted mainly of words she had not become sufficiently fluent to string into sentences.[10]

On her family visits, Lillian witnessed first hand the dire results of

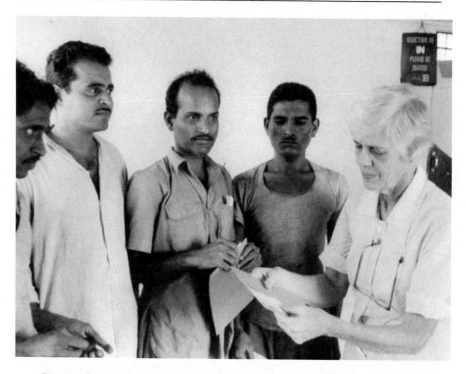

"My mother went into the Peace Corps when she was sixty-eight," quipped Billy Carter in 1976. "My one sister is a motorcycle freak, my other sister is a Holy Roller evangelist and my brother is running for president. I'm the only sane one in the family" (courtesy Peace Corps).

exploding birthrates in a developing country. "The only thing those people had, the only outlet from work, was sex," she explained in a letter, when describing the households she entered. "I would go to the homes where a family—a mother and father and five children—lived in one room, ate, cooked, slept, everything, and had sex right there."[11] On these visits, Lillian would talk to the families about birth control and describe the vasectomy procedure. Though Jimmy Carter writes in *A Remarkable Mother* that these topics were considered taboo by Indians, Lillian and other Peace Corps Volunteers found that most conversations were very much the "anything goes" variety. It was no more taboo to discuss vasectomies than to report to Aloo the state of her hospitalized husband's hemorrhoids, as Lillian did on one memorable occasion. "NOTHING is left unsaid here," Lillian wrote to her family.[12]

And despite the fact that she was in their country to help make sure more of them weren't born, Lillian didn't take long to fall in love with the children of Vikhroli. "Tiny children run up to me," she wrote home, "and hold out their little hands for me to kiss."[13] She recalled a bittersweet experience early in her service when, on her walk home from Kendra, as she dodged cows and goats along the dirt road in ninety degree heat, "a little girl ran to me and handed me a flower. When I stopped to speak to her, about twenty children gathered around to listen to me talk. They are so precious." Yet because most of these children were naked, the effects of their poor diet could be seen all the more plainly in their thin arms and distended bellies.[14] When her family suggested they could send Christmas presents for her to distribute to these children where she saw fit, Lillian had to regretfully decline. "I'd love to have a few toys to give," she wrote back, "but for all the poor, it's just impossible.... They are too poor to eat, much less have a toy." Besides which, if each and every child couldn't have a toy, she would never be happy giving them out to a lucky few.[15]

Lillian was just as unprepared for India's caste system as she was for its malnourished children. Despite efforts to democratize Indian society dating back to the Buddha, modern laws making it illegal to discriminate against someone for being a *dalit* or Untouchable, and Mahatma Gandhi's 1932 hunger strike to bring an end to the system, there were and are still societal and mental walls in India between people as stark as those demarcating black from white in Lillian's native south. When the Reverend Martin Luther King, Jr. went to India with his wife Coretta in 1959, he was surprised to find himself described as one of America's Untouchables. "I started thinking about the fact," he said in a sermon at Ebenezer Baptist Church in Atlanta the year before Lillian started her Peace Corps training. "And I said to myself, Yes, I am an untouchable, and every Negro in the United States of America is an untouchable.'"[16]

Many belonging to India's affluent society were still as blinkered to the problems of inequality as those in the United States. Lillian had come to India on a mission of goodwill among people not likely to have cared how many dresses she bought each year or how much gold jewelry she owned. But such was the object of the questions she fielded all too often from ladies in Vikhroli. She claimed they could not believe that a wealthy American woman bought only four dresses per year, as she assured them she did. According to Lillian, they even asked her why she didn't wear any of her jewelry, prompting her to point out that where she came from, it was not appropriate to wear jewelry and fashionable dresses when serving the poor. Aloo seems to have further irked Lillian when she shared with her the news that Vikhroli was to be honored by a visiting maharaja. Lillian could not have cared less. As she remarked in a letter to her family, "I'm much more interested in the people"—the workers and widows and their children. "Wherever I go," she wrote gleefully, "a crowd gathers." She was so interested in the rank and file that she had put some noses out of joint by the casual way in which she greeted the Godrej brothers. "Everyone was amazed because I simply said, 'How do you do?'" she wrote home. "They all bow and scrape to [the Godrej family]. I won't ever do that." When Mrs. Godrej, obviously with respect and the assumption that Lillian might be some sort of Mrs. Godrej back home in Plains, asked her her opinion of how to improve the Godrej factories, Lillian reported she had curtly replied, "I couldn't tell what improvements the factories needed, as I had never been in any in America except my own." However she did perk up at Mrs. Godrej's other question. How, she asked Lillian, did she think she could be best utilized in Vikhroli? Though Lillian had already been placed by Aloo in the welfare center, Mrs. Godrej must have been a discerning person to have determined that Lillian had far more expertise and energy than could be justified by sending her on family planning visits and looking after children. (In fact, in one of her letters home, Lillian suggests that perhaps there was a bit of jealousy on the part of Aloo, who held the prestige of having Lillian under her supervision, and did not want to lose her to the clinic or some other part of the Godrej operation; on at least one occasion, Lillian hints, Aloo didn't convey to her a request for assistance from the clinic, which Aloo was to have shared with Mabel to share with Lillian.) Lillian told Mrs. Godrej she believed she could most be of help to Dr. Ghanshyam D. Bhatia, the thirty-year-old Hindu who ran the Vikhroli clinic, whom she had just met. To Lillian's surprise and gratefulness, Mrs. Godrej arranged for her to work with Dr. Bhatia on an as-needed basis.[17]

Years later, Dr. Bhatia emphasized just how much he needed the help. "I was handling 200 to 300 patients a day," he recalled. From the start he found Lillian to be an ideal assistant. Though some people wondered that a grandmother with white hair would be able to handle a needle as dexterously as required, Dr. Bhatia had nothing but admiration for Lillian's technique. Her hand, he insisted, "was steady as a rock." Besides giving injections, Lillian dressed and sutured wounds, helped with physiotherapy and gave infrared ray treatments, and was even responsible later on, according to Dr. Bhatia, for organizing the clinic's dispensary. "In the original plan," he recalled, "the dressing room [for wounds] and the room for giving injections were placed together. She said, no, this won't do," and rearranged their placement for better infection control. (The Godrej family would lean on her again in future for advice during planning for a new hospital.)

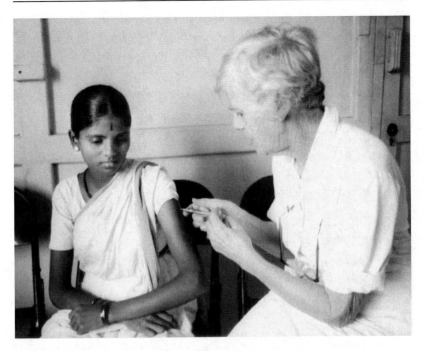

In just one day at Dr. Bhatia's clinic in Vikhroli, Lillian gave injections to four hundred children, her hand "steady as a rock," said Dr. Bhatia. "I have never been so happy," Lillian wrote to her family (courtesy Peace Corps).

Lillian would also urge Dr. Bhatia to set up an emergency room for patients in critical condition.[18]

Lillian had a gift for calming patients who were distressed. As in rural Georgia, her compassion was fueled by outrage over injustices inflicted on the helpless. Though coerced vasectomies were by no means the norm—Carol Stahl, who assisted at more than five hundred operations, knew of no such coercion, noting that men were lining up for the procedure—Lillian claimed that many of the patients at the Godrej clinic were not always there because they wanted to be. And she was disgusted by the way she saw some of these patients, many fearful of the knife, being treated by the surgeon. She noticed that when the clinic staff had completed vasectomy operations they were given soft drinks, while the patients were sent on their way with nothing. The surgeon, whom she confessed she immediately disliked for his brusque manner with the men, angered her by instructing her, with what she heard as sarcasm, "to PAMPER the patients." This, she explained, also sarcastically, "means being kind and holding their hands, and talking to them." She confessed that she frequently found herself mumbling in the surgeon's direction, "Stinking S.O.B." She made sure to always remain in the operating room with the patients. "At least I could console them!" Lillian told her family. She did so by putting cooling damp cloths or just her hands on their heads or murmuring soothing words in Marathi or Gujurati as she massaged their backs.[19]

By March, Lillian was still mostly working with the Kendra children, and she was also working on something she never thought, back in Georgia, would be among her tasks in India: a puppet show. The show was actually her own idea—a way for her to express family planning principles via a medium that most Indians would relate to, puppet shows being part of Indian street and religious fairs since ancient times, and one that would allow her to use her limited Hindi in a creative way, by memorizing and then taping set phrases to use in tandem with the action. The plot involved an argument between a husband and wife, puppets she manipulated in a little stage. The setting allowed Lillian to insert very frank statements about birth control which she or her interlocutors might have had trouble sharing face to face. Her performance was clearly as entertaining as it was informative, because before long she was putting on her show for large audiences— up to two thousand at one time, according to one of her letters.[20]

The puppets were at least a creative outlet for her amid a good deal of routine work and even drudgery. She wrote home that "I've quit being sensitive about Aloo asking me to work & not asking Mabel—It's because I'm so willing & she knows I'll get it done." "I work hard at everything she tells me to do," Lillian added in another note, "but can't cater to her trivial wishes." Yet later that month she wrote home with great joy that she had helped Dr. Bhatia at the clinic the entire day, giving injections to almost four hundred children. "I am so tired," she exclaimed, "and REFRESHED!" Such a day was as yet a rarity so long as she was, in essence, trapped into making posters, selling toothbrushes ("Why? toothbrushes? I think they have a deal to get percent of profit from sale"), filing cards in the clinic and looking after children thanks to her own stalwart energy and eagerness to please.[21]

As she negotiated her time between Kendra and the clinic, Lillian was also working hard to fit into the community. "You'll all think I'm nuts," she wrote, "when I get home and say 'Aaehaa! Selah! Jao!' and nod my head, but it will be a natural thing for me by then."[22]

Toward the end of March, she attended what she called a "God Festival" (possibly Rama Navami, the birthday of the god Rama) with Dr. and

Mrs. Bhatia. Dr. Bhatia remembers taking her to many such festivals as well as Indian weddings, events in which Lillian showed greater interest throughout her stay. In one letter home, Lillian wrote about entering a temple for the first time, in which the figure of the deity was placed on the floor surrounded by marigolds. "I went up to the god, bowed, and dropped a coin into a plate." On the way out, "I had to salaam to everybody present," a respectful gesture she enjoyed giving and receiving.[23] Later that year, she attended one of Mumbai's greatest festivals, Ganpati, the celebration of the elephant-headed god Ganesha. (Perhaps knowing he was the god who removed obstacles, Lillian paid him extra attention.) Colored and gilded plaster figures of the god were decorated with marigolds and given offerings of fruit and ghee before being taken in gala procession down to the Arabian Sea and placed in the water to dissolve. "I've spanned two civilizations," Lillian quipped in a letter home, having first read all the Georgia newspapers used as packing for her care package from Plains before allowing red and yellow dots to be painted on her forehead and between her eyes in preparation for joining her friends at the Ganpati temple.[24] She celebrated Diwali, India's festival of lights, with the Bhatias in Mumbai, well aware what an honor had been shown her to be invited to take *darshan* and offer prayers with her friends. She wrote home that she and the Bhatias "went to an eight-hundred-year old temple to give flowers to the god, then were allowed to enter the presence of the Swami, who gave me a sip of water from the Ganges River." The attention she drew as one of the few foreigners present for the festivities bothered her only to the degree that she wanted to be accepted as just another member of the community. As usual, though, she found something amusing about the situation. "I watched the fireworks," she noted, "while everyone else watched me!"[25]

One of the reasons Lillian so easily made friends among her Indian neighbors was the concern she showed for learning the customs and doing as her friends did, even when this meant eating something she didn't like or, in one example that amused her, taking part in a festival celebrating male virility despite the fact she had been sent to India to promote family planning. She learned that only Muslim and Christian Indians buried their dead; Hindus cremated theirs and cast the ashes into the holy Ganges, while Parsis left theirs in places like Mumbai's "Tower of Silence" to be devoured by vultures. She finally got the hang of eating only with her right hand (the left was used only after going to the toilet), and any time she had an opportunity to watch some dish being made, or how ordinary Indians lived, she seized it—learning how to grind coconut chutney, for example, though this was not something she was likely to have to put into practice herself. "She wasn't interested in tourism," said D. M. Parekh, head of the dyeing and printing factory who met her at this time. "She just wanted to know how human beings live."[26]

She soon reached that level of immersion in another culture where it seems not just difficult but absurd to describe the experience to people back home. When her letters describing how her Indian friends worshiped made their way to Plains, Lillian received a note from a church group there asking her to write about religion in India for a Sunday school class. She hardly knew where to begin. "Good grief!" Lillian wrote. "What on earth would I say? These forty different gods are the same as mine!" Later on, she told her family that "somehow, Hinduism is seeping into my dormant mind, and I know that, somehow, this is my REINCARNATION!" Information like that may well have been more than the Plains Sunday school class could have digested. But it shows that Lillian had already discovered more than her reincarnation—she realized that part of her heart was already Indian, even as in Georgia she had felt it to be partly African. Her wish to be a part of a community of color was becoming, at least in theory, closer to reality.[27]

According to Lillian, Dr. Bhatia was one of those people who seemed too perfect to imagine going to the bathroom after the manner of lesser mortals. He was "the most enlightened person I know," she said, and she listened to him on most subjects. But she couldn't agree with him on what would eventually become a matter of chronic contention between them. "Dr. Bhatia warned me again today," she wrote in June, "that I'm getting too wrapped up in the patients." As he told Lillian, "sometimes he wished I hadn't come to India, because when I leave, so many could not understand."[28]

Dr. Bhatia could just as well have told her that getting too close could break her own heart, too. One patient she came to love was a child who first arrived at the clinic in April, whom she described as "the sweetest little dirty, cross-eyed boy." He had no clothes except a patched pink shirt, and he was always ill. He rarely spoke, but they communicated through her care for him. Lillian clipped his nails and cleaned him up, treated him for the mumps and the boils on his face, and made sure his name was placed on the list to have his eyes surgically straightened. She gave him shots each week, noting with approval that he never whimpered, though sometimes tears would roll down his cheeks during injections, and she always had small gifts of food or old Christmas cards for him, which he treasured. "I wish he had a toy," she told her family, "he's never seen one." When monsoon season arrived, Lillian bought the boy an umbrella, and for a few minutes this child to whom no one had ever paid much attention was the cynosure of the village. "About forty folks gathered around him," Lillian reported, "all talking at once, and showing him how to open it."[29]

It was all too brief. A month later, when the boy had still not come for his next appointment, Lillian realized she would never see him again. "I know that he is dead," she wrote, "but I simply cannot bear to face the reality. It is horrid to realize that I will never know the destiny of this child," the burden of whose fate "will always be with me."[30]

Yet far worse than the case of this boy that she had loved and lost was that of a woman whom Lillian never knew at all.

Lillian first saw her in early May. On her way home, she heard what she thought was a snake rattling in the dry reeds alongside the dirt road. Looking closer, she glimpsed a body lying in the grass—that of a filthy, starving woman, ridden with lice and leprosy.[31] Lillian panicked. "I went flying down to the welfare station," she told an interviewer, "to get somebody to help me. And they laughed at me." The woman's situation was, to them, simply her karma, a concept described acidly by V.S. Naipaul: "the distress we see is to be relished as religious theatre."[32] Lillian told Jimmy in later years that the sound of that laughter, over something so far from being funny, would always haunt her. A doctor she spoke to turned out to be as compassionless as the people at Kendra. Not only did he criticize her for meddling in affairs that were not her business, but as Lillian later remembered with amazement, he accused her of being some sort of geriatric operative of the CIA.[33]

Dr. Bhatia, whom she talked to next, already knew about the dying woman. She had infectious leprosy, he explained to Lillian, and at this point could not be helped. It was better to let her die. Perhaps the people at the welfare station were right—feeding her only prolonged the woman's agony—but Lillian couldn't see it that way. For weeks, as she passed by the woman, she did what she could for her. Once she emptied her wallet into the woman's hands. She regularly brought her bread and water or sent it by a little boy from Vikhroli. After watching the woman drag herself, her fingers eaten by disease, her whole body "a solid sore, and ... diarrheahing all over the place," to drink from a mud puddle, Lillian vented her anger and sorrow in a letter. "I'm at a loss," Lillian raged to her family, "wondering what is to be done in a country so hopeless that they let a woman lie by the side of the road to DIE without help." Dr. Bhatia was firm with her. "It's survival of the fittest, Missy," he adjured her; "you are banging your head on a stone wall." Every time she saw the woman, who finally did die at the end of May, Lillian confessed, "something in me dies." This experience was to segue into another encounter with leprosy, one she had to deal with at closer quarters than from the other side of a busy dirt road.[34]

Lillian was helping Dr. Bhatia in mid–May when an eight year old girl was brought into the clinic. She was Lillian's first close-up experience of leprosy. What made the case even more upsetting to her was that the child's parents, according to Lillian, had no interest in getting her treated, preferring—like those who had laughed at the leper woman—that since she could not be cured, she should die. As Lillian recalled, she felt ashamed of herself for the way she almost unconsciously reacted after having been in the room with the girl only a short time. "I've washed my hands," she admitted, "until they're sore." A few days later, at finding a patch of rough skin on her leg, she begged Dr. Bhatia to look at the area, fearing the worst. He rather amusedly told her that it was just dirt.[35]

Not long after she had seen the eight year old, another child, aged eleven and far more ill, was brought into the clinic by her father. She weighed just thirty pounds, Lillian recalled, and was "slung over [her father's] shoulder like a sack of flour." Lillian was making the child comfortable when she found out that she had infectious leprosy, like the woman beside the road. Unlike the woman, there was still a chance for this girl; if it was possible to save her, treatment had to be started immediately.

As the man placed his daughter on a cot in the examination area, Lillian made an excuse to see Dr. Bhatia. She told him about the case, and that she couldn't touch this girl. She wouldn't be able to treat her. Even when Dr. Bhatia reassured her—"You know leprosy isn't transmitted by touching," he said. "Try to treat her. If you can't, I come do it"—Lillian quailed. She also knew how difficult that "I come do it" was for a man who had hundreds of other patients to see. So she returned to the examination room and through sheer force of will treated the girl, remembering that the doctor had told her that what he needed was a "useful, intellectual nurse," who would carry out her responsibilities in a businesslike and efficient manner. This she tried to do. But after the patient left, "I washed my hands and washed them again," Lillian recalled. The next week, as she gave the girl her injections, she felt the same stabbing fear of catching the disease herself; she scrubbed her hands and rinsed them in alcohol.[36]

Lillian described in an interview many years later how one day she saw that her fears were not just pointless, but were not helping the child, who she could see was starving not only for medical care but for physical affection. In interviews and in her letters home she was matter-of-fact about this transformation. But with her son Jimmy, Lillian shared a more personal account, which he captured in a poem, *Miss Lillian Sees Leprosy for the First Time*:

> When I nursed in a clinic near Bombay,
> a small girl, shielding all her leprous sores,
> crept inside the door. I moved away,
> but then the doctor called, "You take this case!"
> First I found a mask, and put it on,
> quickly gave the child a shot and then,
> not well, I slipped away to be alone
> and scrubbed my entire body red and raw.
>
> I faced her treatment every week with dread
> and loathing—of the chore, not the child.
> As time passed, I was less afraid,
> and managed not to turn my face away.
> Her spirit bloomed as sores began to fade.
> She'd raise her anxious, searching eyes to mine,
> to show she trusted me. We'd smile and say
> a few Marathi words, then touch and hold
> each other's hands. And then love grew between
> us, so that when I kissed her lips,
> I didn't feel unclean.[37]

Her initial response to the leprosy case aside, Lillian, according to Dr. Bhatia, was completely lacking in fear. This fearlessness extended to what she was willing to do to care for her patients in acts which crossed the caste lines that few Indians were willing or able to breach. One of her associates and friends, a male nurse named Raja, was astonished to witness the extent to which Lillian would go to ease patients' discomfort and ensure that they and the clinic were clean. He recalled the time when a patient was admitted with diarrhea so severe he had soiled his pants and the floor. Raja and Lillian removed the man's pants and she asked the cleaner, the *jamadar*, to wash them. The *jamadar* was a sweeper but clearly this was not among the jobs he believed it was his to do, and he refused. Lillian rolled up her sleeves and, with the patient taken in hand by Raja, set to work to wash the dirty clothes and the floor herself. Ashamed at seeing this, the *jamadar* relented. "You see," Raja said, "there was no work she considered degrading."[38]

Fearlessness and kindness extended to the company Lillian kept. As in Plains, when she had spent what to many white residents of the town may have seemed too much time with black families, Lillian set tongues wagging in Vikhroli by openly consorting with people that nobody else wanted anything to do with. "There I was in the living room," she wrote in a letter describing one of her "Untouchable" dinner parties at 13/6, "with a peon, a driver, a labor official, and two staff members. I hate to think what the folks downstairs thought was going on—people here don't even speak to peons, drivers, or any lower caste if they can help it." It's clear she didn't really care what the people downstairs thought, and word got out that 13/6 was a place you could go and be treated with the same respect as your alleged betters. Lillian was especially touched when a young driver came to visit her, albeit with the utmost secrecy: as a man of the servant class, he was never supposed to pay a social call on a person like Lillian. The young man's wife had put him up to it, "so she could see the 'American house,'" Lillian wrote. Lillian loved to oblige. It was like Plains all over again, when her black friends dared not come in the front door, but this time she could do as she pleased. Not only was she able to welcome people who in the American south would have been treated as "coloreds," but she gladly broke the rules of caste distinctions held so dear by upper caste society in India. "I've completely fallen in love with the Indian people I know," she wrote. "Not the bosses—but the masses."[39]

There is no doubt that Lillian was in complete agreement, at least in theory, with the need for birth control in India. Every day, she said, she saw "little babies as small as mice, no food, no clothes, no nothing.... I'm sure my God doesn't want babies hatched like fish!" She had admittedly had some souring experiences visiting families who didn't trust her and wouldn't let their children have the milk, fruit or medicines she offered. On one visit, Lillian recalled, the family "practically forced me out."[40]

The occasional negative home visit was to be expected, but many were positive. What turned her against advising men to have vasectomies was her role in what she believed was the ruin of one man's life. According to her account, having convinced a Vikhroli father to undergo a vasectomy, Lillian heard that three weeks later a smallpox epidemic had claimed his two sons, leaving the father devastated. "Over there [in India]," she said, "unless you have boys, you're nothing.... And I saw that man just almost lose his mind."[41]

She was so troubled by his despair that she knowingly went against what she had been trained to do in Chicago. When she talked to men about family planning she told them privately that they could avoid vasectomy by making their wives undergo tubal ligation. At least then, she reasoned, since that procedure was reversible (as was vasectomy, it should be noted), if an epidemic claimed their boys they could try to have more. This was not advice that would help reduce India's birth rate crisis, but it did help individual men. As Lillian never saw people except as individuals, each with their own set of separate issues just as important as (if not more than) those of the aggregate, she simply ignored the bigger picture. Along with it, Lillian scoffed at Mrs. Gandhi's grand plan, which she early on decided was just politics as usual. As far as she was concerned, Indira Gandhi wasn't really all that concerned about what happened. "Mrs. Gandhi herself, cares nothing for the poor," Lillian asserted. "She's just a politician"—heavy criticism indeed coming from a lifelong political animal like Lillian Carter. One of Lillian's more public criticisms of Indira Gandhi's government was that food aid sent to India by the United States was nullified by graft on the part of the officials who were supposed to ensure that it was delivered to those who needed it. "The things we send them never get to the poor," Lillian claimed baldly in an interview years later. "They're divided among the big shots in the government." However Carol Stahl has a different take on this. "I was in a group of Westerners and middle (not upper) class Indians," she recalls. "The people of India did not like the wheat the U.S. sent—it wasn't hard enough or something. Someone (a Westerner) expressed concern that the wheat from the U.S. might have mold or rot because it was just dumped loose into the hold of ships, not bagged or contained, and did anyone have an opinion on whether it was safe to eat? The Indians laughed and said that because the grain was loose, it had to be shoveled out of the ship. Did we really think that the very poor men who did that kind of hot, hard manual labor left their work to go find a toilet to relieve themselves? Why worry about mold?"[42]

Sometimes the struggle to balance what were two different lives was just too exhausting. Finding herself unable to meet the most basic needs of privacy, except in the bathroom, began to tell on Lillian's nerves. She was discovering in the crowded suburbs of India's largest city, to quote Mumbai native Suketu Mehta, that "the greatest luxury of all is solitude,"[43] and her temper flared, sometimes at Mabel. "I have to pray all the time," she wrote home in March, "to keep from pushing Mabel out the window—thank goodness they have steel bars over them." In April, she confessed that "God is letting me stand [Mabel] a lot better, but I got to where I really considered pushing her down the steps."[44] This was typical Lillian exaggeration—back in Plains, she was known to "fire" her longtime housekeeper, Lillian Pickett, who, understanding Lillian all too well, would sit in the front yard for a while, then return to the house, where the outburst was not mentioned and life went on as before. Lillian and Mabel were very different women from very different backgrounds and sets of priorities. In

India, Mabel wouldn't walk, even short distances, if she could catch a ride in a car, and she wouldn't focus on Hindi—indeed, Lillian claims Mabel tried to dissuade her from pursuing Hindi studies. She didn't like company at 13/6 in the evening, which meant Lillian had to teach her English classes to Indian men at offsite locations. Lillian believed that walking to work, participating in Indian life and language, helped her become more Indian herself. "My contact with the people here is so much *wider* and deeper if I walk," she wrote. When she returned to the apartment to find the very American Mabel continually present, frustrations arose for both women. "My grandmother was not easy to warm up to," says Scott Yewell. "She'd been a military nurse—an excellent nurse—but she was old school and rigid and opinionated," which was where she and Lillian definitely parted company. "They liked each other," he adds, "but it was more a case of tolerating each other." Carol Stahl claims that Mabel was "very overshadowed" by Lillian, but she did not lack spunk. This is clear from a remark Mabel made to a reporter when she and Lillian visited ten years after their return from India. Asked if anything had changed between them, Mabel said, "We're the same old bitches." As Lillian wrote to Anne Yewell Ashton, Mabel's granddaughter, after Mabel's death, "I really loved her—& she did me—but we have laughed over the times when we yelled at one another in our house—getting on each others' nerves. I'm sure she had the worst of it."[45]

While most of the frustration Lillian experienced was due to her unsatisfactory work situation, some of it came from doubts about the viability of what she was doing. Lillian had been receiving worried letters from home. She had been too truthful about the conditions in which she lived every day—the death and disease, the lack of adequate food, walking miles in the heat in her bare feet, and the debilitating frustration that she couldn't be more useful. Knowing only this side of the story, Lillian's children were alarmed to the point where Jimmy urged his mother to come home. Lillian's worst fear was not so much that she might catch a disease or drop from exhaustion but that she had come to India for reasons that were not as pure as she had believed. "I left all personal worries behind me, and am in another world," she wrote, "where my worries are not personal, but of such huge proportions that it takes more than just me to overcome them." Exchanging one set of problems—personal ones—for the weight of the world was not so fair a trade.[46]

As her dissatisfaction and doubt reached critical mass, Lillian needed a place where she could discreetly unburden her soul, and through perhaps her kindest Indian friend, she found it. The Godrej family's head gardener,

Mr. Vinod, was keeping her and Mabel in constant supply of fresh flowers, often driving Lillian to the greenhouse so she could get a first look at newly opened exotic blooms. He also kept the women stocked with fresh vegetables, improving a diet which was either feast when canned goods arrived from family overseas or famine when they lived on chapattis and rice. In turn, Lillian was teaching Mr. Vinod's little daughter, Madhavi, to read, and was already giving her books, one of the signal indications of Lillian's respect and affection. Perhaps Mr. Vinod told Lillian about the rose garden he had planted on a hill near the apartment house. Always disliking public displays of personal faith, Lillian made the garden a kind of private outdoor chapel. She would sit hidden among the rocks "and talk to Jesus," as she told an interviewer, "just as if he was in the room. I told him, 'I would never have come over here if you hadn't brought me, and you'll have to do something.'" The something she wanted done through divine intervention was that she not have to work in Kendra any more but as full-time nurse in the Godrej clinics. "I knew nothing about the new medicines," she admitted, "but I never forgot how to take a temperature; I never forgot how to give injections." Most of all, nursing was her calling—it was inextricably tied to her heart and her compassion, and where these were employed Lillian Carter was a force to be reckoned with. Even in her darkest hours, she was never in any doubt "that God is looking at me." And so, as she wrote to her children, it was to Heaven that she now turned for a deciding answer. "'Come on, God,'" she demanded, "'this is your problem!'"[47]

The answer came toward the end of June, though from a more earthly source of benevolence. "Mrs. Godrej asked me when I was going back to my school work," she wrote home, "and I said, 'Whenever you say,' and she said, 'No—from now on, your work is at the Clinic with Dr. Bhatia.'" Lillian captured her bliss in six simple words: "I have never been so happy."[48]

When he took her on as his full-time nurse, Dr. Bhatia made a first aid kit for Lillian containing "all kinds of medicines for itch, boils, malnutrition, even a triangular cloth to put over heads with lice," Lillian recalled. It was to be used when help was needed outside the clinic. Little did the doctor realize that Lillian would extend "outside" well beyond the boundaries of Godrej Industries.

When her day's work at the clinic was done, Lillian had to walk more than a mile along a dirt road—the same one where she had found the dying leper woman—to reach the apartment she shared with Mabel. Along the way, "I would meet children who wanted me to do something," Lillian said.

"Maybe they had some lumps, or something, or bad sore legs. And I'd meet women who would beg me to do something." Because she always carried the first aid kit with her, she spent a lot of her time between the clinic and home fixing people up, she wrote, "right there in the middle of the road." The problem was, these were not the children of Godrej employees but of the people who lived in the grass and mud huts on the hills. As a Peace Corps Volunteer assigned to the Godrej complex, Lillian couldn't and shouldn't have been doing anything for anybody except employees. She knew the clinic was only for those who were. But as her helpfulness became known, requests from the non–Godrej people increased, and soon exceeded what she was able to do with her first aid supplies. So she overstepped another invisible status line and arranged a meeting with one of the Godrej brothers who, as she told her family, were so rich you didn't go to them, they summoned you.[49]

Lillian asked Mr. Godrej point-blank for money and for permission to give medical aid to the poor outside the walls of the complex who requested and needed it. "He thought I was crazy," she recalled. Nobody had that much money, Mr. Godrej told her—echoing the attitude of the Indian government—that would be necessary to take care of so many poor people. Frustrated, Lillian began to cry. "I cannot stand this any longer," she told him, and that if he didn't assist her she would have to tender her resignation, since she couldn't see these sick people every day and not help them. Mr. Godrej asked her to reconsider, but eventually her threats—and her tears—seemed to work, because he relented to a certain degree. "He told me that if I could get [Dr. Bhatia] to see more people, and if we could get medicine, and if I would stand by the gate and only let people through who I felt were sick enough, he would permit it," she recalled. It was only half the battle, as she now had to enlist the sympathies of Dr. Bhatia.[50]

Lillian went to Dr. Bhatia and laid the charm on thick. "They love flattery," she said later, meaning Indian men, "oh my, I think all men do." Lillian told Dr. Bhatia that if she should have the misfortune to contract cholera or leprosy after she returned to Georgia, she hoped he would allow her to come back to Vikhroli to be treated solely by him. Dr. Bhatia knew better, pointing out that there were far more advanced medical facilities in the United States than in India. Oh no, Lillian averred, that simply wasn't so; they didn't know a thing compared to him. "I told him how beautiful his wife was," she recalled, "what a cute little daughter he had, and after a while he was just beaming." Then she dropped the bombshell about her meeting with Mr. Godrej. "The doctor hit the ceiling," she recalled, "because he was seeing between two and three hundred patients a day already." Lillian's unremitting flattery, however, and her assurances that her help would ease the additional workload, softened the blow, and nurse and doctor came to an agreement. For any woman or child from outside who presented themselves at the gate, Lillian would be called to determine the seriousness of their condition and authorize their admittance.[51]

But opening the clinic gates had a decided downside. Though a well-off woman back home, Lillian had little money in India. Of the small set amount she received each month from the Peace Corps, between taking care of her own needs and her generosity to the villagers she had very little left for anything else, and she wasn't allowed to take money from her family. This Peace Corps rule was there to be broken, however; according to Jimmy Carter, his mother cashed a personal check and gave a box filled with rupees to Dr. Bhatia to use for purchasing more drugs. Lillian then wrote to Jimmy, pleading that he persuade drug companies to send her any surplus medicines and any samples they had, which he did.[52] And during her increasingly sleepless nights, she came up with what she called "the craziest scheme you ever heard of. I was learning," she said, with manifest pride, "to steal and tell lies for those people."[53]

She confessed in an interview a decade later:

> We had two drug salesmen who sold American drugs and we had Lilly's drug company, it was about ten miles from us, and about twenty miles on the other side was Parke-Davis, and every Monday morning one or the other came. Parke-Davis's man came on a Monday, and I told him a long tale about how much we helped the poor and how I know Mr. Parke and Mr. Davis very well, and if you would give me some samples, I would write both of them what wonderful work you're doing. And I was so serious he swallowed it. He gave me the samples he had for that day.[54]

When the man from Lilly paid a call, Lillian enlisted the prestige of her senatorial son, telling the salesman that Jimmy had attended school with Eli Lilly's son (or grandson—she left it vague), and that they were quite good friends. "I soon had cabinets full of medicine samples," she recalled, and the extra people she and Dr. Bhatia treated could have medicines just as the Godrej employees did.[55] Adding more patients to the daily queue and scamming drug salesmen to get medicines for them added more hours to Lillian's already long days, and Dr. Bhatia didn't hesitate to give her all the work and then some that she could handle. As Mrs. Godrej recalled in later years, "Lillian's outstanding quality, I think, was her devotion to duty." Though she could often see that Lillian was tired and needed rest, she would never take it, even when urged. "She insisted on carrying on," said Mrs. Godrej.[56] It was easy for her to do, because Lillian wanted to help everyone—she was never happier than when fully engaged in solving the problems, health-related or otherwise, of other people. When Dr. Bhatia sent her and Raja to examine the eyes of all five thousand Godrej workers, Lillian was thrilled. It wasn't just because she could test her medical skills in a far bigger way than she ever had before, or that this was more proof that Dr. Bhatia's trust in her was growing, though these were significant milestones. When the doctor had once described her as an "efficient nurse," what might have sounded to another person like an everyday affirmation was to Lillian an occasion that, as she wrote her family, "will stand out in my future as pillars of fire."[57] The best part of treating all the Vikhroli workers, she explained, was being able to meet and interact personally with them. Among these five thousand men, "there are hundreds," she said, "who have never before had any contact with an educated or a kind, understanding soul." She wanted to make sure the men had healthy eyes, but she also wanted to be to them that kind and understanding soul.[58]

At this time, one of Lillian's Indian friends gave her a copy of *The Art of Living*, one of several books written by Swami Chinmayananda. Born Balakrishna Menon in 1916, the swami had been active in the movement to free India from British rule; he had also worked as a journalist. On a visit to the severely strict Himalayan holy man, Swami Sivananda, for an assignment to write a piece criticizing Hindu monks, Menon was so moved by the swami he became a monk himself. Dr. Bhatia's brother was a devoted follower of the now famous former reporter, describing to Lillian how he had attained monkhood and the name Swami Chinmayananda Saraswati ("filled with the bliss of pure consciousness"). Lillian eventually read all of the swami's books, but she was especially fond of *The Art of Living*. In this book, the swami ranked the three classes of men: those who labored for their own selfish ends, those who worked selflessly toward an ideal, and those men of achievement who, Lillian explained, "are not after mere pleasures nor do they aspire to reform the world, but perform their duties finding peace and fulfillment in their activity. The latter seems to be my aim at this point." Lillian's book-giving friend saw this perhaps even more clearly than she did. "To Amma [Mother] Carter," he wrote, "who has travelled thousands of miles to our ancient land to seek fulfillment in the evening of her present life. A step towards her journey to reach the Kingdom of Heaven within herself."[59]

In the crowded, chaotic, and often heart-breaking rooms of the clinic, Lillian Carter had finally reached that kingdom, and added a fourth degree to the swami's classes of men: that of *Aai*—Mother.

CHAPTER 7

Coming Home

For Lillian's second Christmas in Vikhroli, she and other Peace Corps Volunteers were sent to Goa to celebrate the holidays together. On Christmas Day, when the young Volunteers left to check out Goa's nightlife, Lillian descended to the hotel kitchens "and just took over the supervision of preparing the Christmas dinner," she wrote her family. In all, she and the cooks prepared a dozen turkeys with all the trimmings—food in quality and quantity none of them had enjoyed for months. When the Volunteers returned to find such a feast waiting for them, "they actually applauded," Lillian wrote home, which "made my day complete. I hope your Christmas was as happy as mine!"[1]

Back in Vikhroli, Lillian had a more simple celebration. She had already set up a Christmas tree, thanks to Mr. Vinod. He gave her a miniature pine, the sight of which almost brought her to tears. But she assured her family that her emotions were in check. "I will NOT give way to my feelings," she wrote. "I'm going to put something on [the tree] for decoration, and put my gifts under it (I hid them in my suitcase to relieve my temptation), and I WILL celebrate Christmas!"[2]

Two days into 1968, Lillian thanked everyone back home for their presents but with her gratitude came an apology, because she had redistributed everything to her Indian friends. "I realized that their kindness to me was the one thing that sustains me," she explained to her family, "and I gave all my gifts away, one by one. I couldn't help it. I had already had the joy of receiving them, and I just had no other way to pass that joy along to these people who have come to mean so much to me."[3] Her Christmas present to Mabel was one of the more precious items from her Georgia food parcel—"it was the only thing she wanted," Lillian explained, "a jar of mustard!"[4] She had even parted with the one expensive purchase she had allowed herself during her time in India, a cashmere shawl she'd found in Goa. A patient had come into the clinic, very ill with pneumonia. Lillian couldn't bear to see the man shivering in his thin shirt and had wrapped her shawl around him. Having been treated, he departed wearing the shawl. She wrote it off as another joy to pass along—and as she told her family, "Material things have lost all meaning for me."[5]

Lillian's circle in Vikhroli was not the sole beneficiary of her sharing, nor was Christmas her only season for doing so. Gabe and Ruth Ross, who had been so helpful to Lillian during their training in Chicago, had managed to argue themselves out of being posted in Mumbai with such success that the Peace Corps had instead sent them to a remote village nearly two hundred miles away. Shortly after getting settled into 13/6, somehow Lillian obtained the Rosses' address, and it wasn't too long, as Gabe Ross recalls, before he and Ruth began receiving care packages from her. Lillian depended on her packages from Plains as much for moral as physical support; she evidently felt that Gabe and Ruth might need much the same. Most of the books she sent to the Rosses were paperback novels, Gabe remembers, "with a brief note attached. The assumption was that some of these had come from her family. She'd finished reading them and was passing them on."[6] But one of the packages contained a book of more than ordinary quality, Lebanese author Khalil Gibran's greatest work, *The Prophet*. This was not a volume sent to Lillian but one she had carefully packed in her suitcase when she left Plains, and it had taken nearly two frustrating months to reach her in Vikhroli. The day of arrival was treated like a gala event. "I was so happy to see the books I had in it, 'Kim' and 'The Prophet,'" she had written to her family in February 1967. "I just held them close to me and walked around. God bless 'The Prophet'—I can read it over and over and find something new each time."[7] Now this cherished book took another journey, arriving in the little village where Gabe and Ruth were living. "It was inscribed by her," says Gabe, "'I hope you love this as I have.'"[8] As the Rosses would have read when they opened *The Prophet*, "You give but little when you give of your possessions," says Gibran's Al-Mustafa to the people of seaside Orphalese. "It is when you give of yourself that you truly give."[9]

Lillian's letters home are so often about her work in the clinic that it comes as a surprise that she did anything in India that wasn't related to nursing—that she and Mabel went to the Arabian Sea, for example, to wade in the surf and eat ice creams, or that Lillian spent money on anything other than medicines or food for the needy, though in fact she bought books when she could afford them. She did take vacations during her twenty-one months of service, and while each trip was openly celebrated in her letters home as an opportunity to get away from Mabel, Lillian was already eager to expand her horizons beyond Vikhroli. Her first trip away was spent at the old Raj-era hill station of Matheran, to get to which she had to take a romantic if vertiginous train ride from Mumbai. She was "the only American among the Indians," she wrote her family, "and I pretended I was in an Alfred Hitchcock movie, going toward an intriguing destination as the little train went up and up, around and around the mountain for hours, with its eery [sic] whistle shrilling around every curve."[10]

It was now, when she was away from the demands and the adrenaline of the clinic, that Lillian realized how completely exhausted she was. For a few days, she did nothing but relax. She was so taken with the green hills, refreshing to the eye after the brown flatness of the coast, that she claimed she could sit in her room at the Lords Central Hotel watching for hours as storms swept through, lightning flashing and thunder booming. And when the clouds cleared, she was delighted to hear monkeys dancing over the rooftops. "They sound like a football team in the attic," she observed, and confided to her family, "This is the laziest I have ever been in my life."[11] But her natural restlessness took over, as it always did when Lillian had to sit somewhere doing nothing. She hired a Hindi teacher to give her lessons in the language that the Peace Corps had failed to offer, only to find that their sessions were mostly taken up by his fascination with her radio, perhaps a by-product of Indira Gandhi's pre-premier role as Minister of Information and Broadcasting and promoter of radio's marvels. "He just sat and listened to it," she wrote, "completely engrossed, until I finally told him to take it with him, and invited him to come back to dinner." When he returned, he had the volume turned all the way up; Lillian promised him he could take it home that night if he switched it off during dinner. It might have been better to have the radio on: during the meal, the tutor freely indulged in burping with histrionic satisfaction. "It is etiquette for middle- and low-class Indians," Lillian explained, "but this is one aspect of their culture I will NOT adopt!"[12]

She never did make much headway in Hindi, and perhaps was glad of it on this occasion, because she just couldn't stay in her room any longer. Through means she doesn't explain, Lillian made social visits to local families. "I had tea with a Hindu couple yesterday," she wrote in one letter. "He and I sat on pots (stools) and watched while she made tea." The table was made of cow dung, she said, as were the floors, and the lady of the house wiped them and the cups with the same cloth, which she held in her toes. But this wasn't what made Lillian object to the meal when it was served. After placing the plates and cups in front of Lillian and her husband, the wife then sat off by herself, which was according to Hindu custom practiced throughout the country and sanctioned by the ancient Hindu epic, the *Mahabarata*. "Of excellent vows, she never eats before I eat, and never bathes before I bathe," says the great prince Bhishma of his devoted wife. "Ever devoted to her lord and ever relying upon her lord, she was ever employed in doing what was agreeable to and beneficial for her lord."[13]

Such regard for the husband's every need was seen as an ideal to emulate, but it was a male ideal increasingly questioned by such female powerhouses as Lady Rama Rau, an Indian aristocrat and feminist. When Lillian heard Lady Rama Rau speak at a family planning meeting in Mumbai, she was jolted out of the boredom such conferences usually evoked in her. Founder of the Family Planning Association of India, Lady Rama Rau had been named president of the International Planned Parenthood Federation in 1963, and she brooked no interference from any man, Indian or otherwise, when it came to the rights of women. At the Mumbai conference that Lillian attended, Lady Rama Rau sat on a panel with male speakers and demanded that the practice of marrying girls off be ended definitively (the discussion had begun with the tamer question of merely raising the legal age for marriage). She desired "to educate the women, provide jobs for them, let them learn something of the world," Lillian reported home. She noted that after saying this, Lady Rama Rau then turned to the male official who represented the Indian government and said, "But, I'll fight any legislation for FORCE, Mister, and you can put that in your pipe, take it to Delhi, and tell them!" Lillian commented approvingly, "Boy, I loved that." When she spoke with Lady Rama Rau later, Lillian asked her if she'd ever heard the English slang word "guts." "Hell, yes!" answered Lady Rama Rau. "I learned it years ago in America."[14]

"Wives [in India] are usually boring," Lillian told her family, precisely because they were not educated "and have to treat their husbands like gods!"[15] For Lillian and for many women, liberation had to begin at home. So as she sat at the cow dung table in Matheran, the husband nervously smiling across from her as the wife sat far away, Lillian refused to eat until the wife came to the table and joined them for the meal. "For the FIRST TIME, she ate with her husband!" Lillian noted. Before leaving the house, she made the couple promise to always eat together, "UNLESS someone else was there!" Strictly speaking, it wasn't quite fair for this foreigner to march into an Indian home to challenge old customs, protected only by the fact she was a guest in the house. But in bringing the woman to the table, Lillian had perhaps established a worthy new custom: that of woman taking her place in equal presence and power beside man. Nobody could accuse that of being presumptuous foreign interference—it was the way the world was turning, more than halfway through the twentieth century.[16]

Two weeks into her stay in Matheran, Lillian had what she called "an exciting adventure." She had somehow met up with a swami who was not only popular but thrillingly handsome, replete with entourage and crowds of followers who treated him like a god. Lillian went to hear him lecture; like anyone else, she walked with him and his disciples and meditated with him. "He is glorious," she wrote home, "with his shaved head, earrings, and flowing yellow robe," which signified renunciation. (By contrast, her favorite back in Mumbai, Swami Chinmayananda, often wore every day clothes.) She noted that while his followers bowed to him, hands abjectly on the swami's feet, "and backing away salaaming, I just said, 'Bye now, see you tonight.'" With obvious delight at this informality the holy man told her, "Bye, OK!" Around this time, Lillian encountered another holy man, this one a kind of saddhu or wandering monk. He gave her his walking stick—a signal honor to bestow, and one which seemed to say that though his journey was done, she still had more "exciting adventures" along the highway of life. To Lillian he was "a prophet," perhaps because he looked at her keenly and declared, "You will write a book before 1969." She doesn't seem to have taken this seriously, and couldn't have suspected that in less than a decade, the many letters she was sending to half a dozen members of her family in America would be gathered together and published in a volume that is still in print over thirty years later.[17]

Lillian was not alone in looking for wisdom in far off and far out places, though as with the Peace Corps, she was older than most who did. This was the decade when young Americans were flocking to Indian ashrams, some in search of truth, others in search of hashish, most trying to find some meaning in a decade that embraced in swift succession the assassinations of President Kennedy, Dr. Martin Luther King, Jr., and Senator Robert Kennedy, against a backdrop of race riots and culture wars. Many were seen both at home and abroad less as pilgrims than sensationalists, wild children of the experimental Sixties, and this was often the case. But Mr. Bhatia's sincere effort to include Lillian in every opportunity to hear Swami Chinmayananda lecture seems to indicate he saw her as very different from most foreigners who came to India to discover themselves. As if she were an Indian lady who had grown lax in her observances, he began to give Lillian lectures of his own: that it was improper to ride with a Muslim (a sad commentary on how endemic the Hindu-Muslim conflict was even for an enlightened man like Mr. Bhatia); or that she not go walking by herself at night. Lillian met most of Mr. Bhatia's expectations with enthusiasm, reading the swami's books and discussing their meaning, attending crowded lectures where she sometimes sat on the ground for hours while the swami held forth on such topics as mind over matter, a teaching that Lillian took to heart when her folded legs began to go numb over three hours.[18] On one memorable occasion, Lillian joined what she claimed was a crowd of 30,000 people—the population of a good-sized town in Georgia—"and listened avidly to [Swami Chinmayananda]." Mr. Bhatia insisted that she join him every night for the swami's lectures, "but I am too old and decrepit," she told her family. "Lordy, I have never been so hurried and pushed about—it's like trying to put Barnum and Baileys Circus in my living room, if you can imagine 30,000 people trying to get on the same train at once."[19] These meetings were physically challenging for her, especially after being awake since dawn and on her feet all day, and though she was accompanied home by "two or three escorts who would not catch me if I were falling (because they are too pure to touch any woman other than their wives)," she gained much from the swami's sessions. Lillian once claimed she went to the lectures just to "listen," and likened some of the experiences to the wrestling matches she had so enjoyed in Columbus. Yet she never denied the power of the swami's message. "He said one thing which I will never forget," she told her family. "'If you are good, be DYNAMICALLY good, don't be passively anything!'" Words like these resonated powerfully for the Peace Corps Volunteer, the nurse who worked for free, the lifelong humanitarian.[20]

Though she knew Mr. Bhatia objected to her wearing of short dresses, Lillian got away with it on one supreme occasion, when she had her first face to face meeting with Swami Chinmayananda. Mr. Bhatia introduced Lillian, who was permitted to take the swami's picture, she wrote home on February 28, 1968, "and [I] even got to chat with him for a few minutes." A photo was then taken of the two of them sitting with the rest of the Discussion Group, eating from plates set on the floor. Lillian is seated at the swami's left, and her legs, bared by her scandalous short dress but tucked as discreetly under its hem as she could manage, are there for all to see. "The greatest part of all, though, was the fact that he looked at me once,"

Lillian wrote, "this is considered the highest honor of all!" Obviously, like the wisest holy men, Swami Chinmayananda was able to excuse certain human failings considered too scandalous by his followers.[21]

Lillian's letters home are more like diary entries than ordinary correspondence. While they do report on her surroundings and circumstances, the weather, her aches and pains and her occasional frustrations with Mabel, with the clinic, with Indian customs and with herself, running throughout is a theme that is just as pervasive as her constant hunger: her loneliness. As much as she valued her privacy, and as much as she would have liked more of it at Apartment 13/6, Lillian needed to be needed. This was a major reason for her switch from family planning work to nursing in the clinic; it was why she made such close and devoted friends out of those who were dependent on her for skilled help and simple compassion. There are few pages of any letter Lillian sent to her family over the years 1966–1968 where she doesn't bare her soul in this manner. Where her food shortage was concerned, the Carters did everything they could to make the situation better by supplementing her diet via care packages. What they couldn't do was transport themselves to Vikhroli. This is why Jimmy Carter was carrying his mother's loneliness around in his head the day he met Vice President Hubert Humphrey in Atlanta in 1968. Humphrey was in Atlanta to visit his friend Marvin Shoob, a supporter of Jimmy Carter's first run for governor of Georgia in 1966. Humphrey had been instrumental in making the Peace Corps into a reality, and having never forgotten Lillian's energy and spunk on the Johnson campaign in Georgia, he was especially pleased to hear that she was serving with the Corps in India. He asked Jimmy where his mother was stationed, and how she was doing. Jimmy answered frankly that his mother had written several times of how alone she felt. He told Humphrey that according to his mother, she had not had a visit from a Peace Corps official since arriving in Vikhroli in December 1967. Jimmy happened to notice that one of Humphrey's aides was writing everything he said on a notepad.[22]

Not long after this encounter, in May, the Peace Corps's Country Director for India drove out to Vikhroli from Mumbai and paid Lillian a visit at her apartment. He said he had received a letter from Vice President Humphrey about her; he didn't reveal its contents, but brought her a bottle of Scotch—having understood that she had been under the weather in Madras, he thought she'd like it. He also offered to send a car for her the following week, to bring her into Mumbai to fill out her termination papers, and promised her a feast afterward. "I'LL HAVE A STEAK DINNER!" Lillian crowed. Until she got home and found out what had really happened,

Lillian was probably just as mystified as the Country Director, who turned to her before he left and asked, "Who the Hell ARE you, Lilly?"[23] As Jimmy Carter points out in his memoir of his mother, "She was a friend, once removed, of Vice President Humphrey."[24]

While it was nice receiving all this attention and help with the onerous government paperwork, perhaps worse than loneliness at this juncture was the imminent approach of Lillian's termination date. "I'm getting nervous about coming home," she confessed in a letter written in late July from Vikhroli, "you know, like worms crawling under my skin. But everyone is so sweet to me at the Clinic—they act like I'm going to die." She couldn't face the thought of leaving them, "these wonderful people for whom I've done so little, but who have done so much for me!" Dr. Bhatia's sadness and his quiet regret were hardest for her to bear. "He has forgotten," she said, "what the others did before I came." This comes as no surprise. Lillian had become a serious asset to the clinic, above and beyond the role she had come to fill. Not only was she a superb assistant for Dr. Bhatia, a tireless worker, an indefatigable learner, and a good friend to the other nurses, but she was loved by her patients. When she had first begun to work with Dr. Bhatia and the surgeons, her interest in each patient, her curiosity about their lives, her effort to get at the root of their problems, was scoffed at, as was the help she extended to the "hut people" in the hills, the dying given up as hopeless, the sick children whose imminent demise even parents did little to avoid, since they were just more mouths to feed, and of course the men who feared themselves unmanned by vasectomies. She brought hope and compassion to people who had rarely known either. Well might Dr. Bhatia wonder how he had managed before she came, and how he would manage after she departed. Lillian had become that higher thing than *memsahib*. She was now, to hundreds of people in and around Vikhroli, *Lily behn*: "our sister Lily." That was definitely an office nobody else could fill.[25]

By August, a month before her departure, Lillian was being entertained, "royally," she wrote home, "and accept every invitation—teas, luncheons, dinners—and, best of all, bridge with the Joglekars." The Joglekars were a couple with whom Lillian spent many relaxing evenings. Like her, they enjoyed good books. Mr. Joglekar regularly gave Lillian copies of classics she had already read but prized all the same, and she gave him her copy of *Gone With The Wind*. (The stereotyped Old South of the David O. Selznick film had captured the Indian imagination and every time a southern-themed movie was screened Lillian's friends wanted her to see it and tell them what she thought, since she came from there.) The Joglekars brought a calm into Lillian's frenetic and worry-filled life that she needed as much as she did the busyness of the clinic. She described for her family one such evening with the Joglekars in mid–March. They had played a hand of bridge, then moved out to the balcony to enjoy the cooling breezes. "Oh, it was so beautiful!" Lillian declared. "There was a full moon, and stars. On the hillside were the little lights twinkling in the huts, and in the distance, the Bay with small boat lights. Sometimes I forget to look at beauty." She was to spend her last weeks in India looking at it as hard as she could.[26]

On the day she and Mabel were to board their flights, a party was given for them at the Grand Hotel in Mumbai. Lillian surprised and delighted those present by appearing in full sari.[27] The male nurse Raja was with Lillian when, after the party was over, and with her outfit changed and her suitcase packed, she whispered to him, "Let's go to the airport." Raja always wondered why she had chosen him to come with her, above all the others who might have been happy to be asked. "Maybe she was sick at the idea of leaving India," he surmised later. "But I think her main idea was to tell me to look after her patients."[28]

Gabe and Ruth Ross were also at the airport to see Lillian off. Though his service, like Ruth's, was done, Gabe had been hired by the Peace Corps as coordinator for the new cadre of Volunteers coming to Maharashtra state. Lillian hugged both, as she always did. "Then she reaches into her pocket and pulls out a wad of rupees," recalls Gabe, "and says 'Take these, I don't need them any more. You need them.' 'No, Lilly,'" Gabe joked, "'I'm no longer working for two cents an hour, I'm working for the Peace Corps and thank you, but we'll be fine.'" Lillian held up the handful of bills. "You take it," she warned Gabe, "or I'm throwing it up in the air and we're going to start a riot!"[29]

Lillian's single suitcase was heavy with gifts and mementos from her friends, and she refused to check it through to Atlanta for fear it might get lost. On arriving at Heathrow Airport, she realized she would have to carry it herself some distance to the next gate. Digging into her pocket, all she could find there was ten cents American money. A porter saw the thin elderly lady struggling with the suitcase and offered to help. Lillian thanked him but admitted she couldn't afford to pay him for his trouble. Knowing Lillian, she probably also told him the whole story of where she had been and what adventures she had been having. Suitably seduced, the porter picked up Lillian's suitcase, took her to her departure gate, checked the bag, and wouldn't take the ten cents she offered, saying, "It would be an honor for me to help you." "She made him give her his name and address," Jimmy Carter wrote, "and her first task when she arrived in Plains was to send him her effusive thanks and perhaps the largest tip he had ever received."[30]

"I saved my best dress to wear home," she wrote in her last letter from India. "I know it will be falling apart by the time I get there, so please don't make fun of me.... I do have one consolation—I'm coming home."[31]

Per their mother's instructions, Gloria Carter Spann and her brothers had been waiting three hours at Atlanta Municipal Airport for her 9:30 p.m. arrival.

The refrigerator of Lillian's house in Plains had been stocked full of everything she liked, as if inspired by a list she had lovingly and longingly

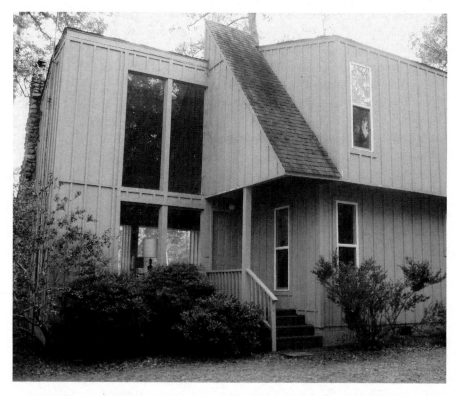

Designed and built as a surprise for Lillian on her return from India in 1968, the Pond House sits on a rise overlooking a fish pond, ringed by Georgia pines alive with squirrels and birds; it still offers a quiet so pure that the flipping of a fish on the pond's still green surface startles like a shot (photograph by the author).

sent home in a letter: "I want a T-bone steak, tossed salad, a biscuit, a good drink ... peach ice cream, a drink, some butter beans ... and a drink...." And waiting in the airport parking lot was a brand new cream-colored Lincoln-Continental, "the kind she'd always wanted," said Gloria.[32]

Everyone was prepared for a joyous and emotional reunion with the woman they had not seen in nearly two years, for whom a one year old granddaughter she had not yet met, Amy Lynn, waited in Plains. "We watched as the plane started unloading," remembered Gloria, "and stood in awe when she appeared at the doorway—so thin, so tired, her dress much too large, and her eyes—searching, searching for a familiar face, but not recognizing any of us." Jimmy got to Lillian first, yet she didn't seem to know who he was. (Nor did she recognize her granddaughter, Kim, who greeted her when she arrived home in Plains. When she asked where Kim was, Sybil Carter had to point out that she was standing right in front of her).[33] This was a scene Lillian had predicted in a letter from a few weeks earlier. "I have nightmares that I will get off the plane and be surrounded by strange white people," she had written.[34] A wheelchair was brought and the frail woman was persuaded to sit in it. As if in a daze, Lillian looked at everyone who passed, then she leapt up and began to follow a man she had seen crossing the lobby. As her children tried to restrain her, Lillian cried out, "Let me go, don't you understand? He's an Indian and he doesn't know anybody here—I've got to stop him and talk to him—he must be homesick and he'll be so glad to see me." Lillian had not only lost thirty-five pounds, and seemed to have aged ten years; it appeared she might have lost her mind as well. But Gloria, Jimmy and Billy suddenly understood. "Our Indian Mother had returned to America," explained Gloria, "but it would be a while yet before our Mother was really home."[35]

Lillian seemed oblivious to the cream-colored Lincoln, though she did see the signs the children made for her homecoming, placing them on fences and trees along the highway to Plains. "WELCOME HOME, GRAND-MAMA.... And when we got to my house, THIS IS GRANDMAMA'S HOUSE. Big signs," she remembered. They brought her through the door she had left unlocked in the fall of 1966. Gloria said, "Look, Mother, we've got everything you want in the refrigerator." Lillian saw the shelves crammed with groceries. "I had craved fried chicken, pimento-and-cheese sandwiches, and chocolate cake, and I hadn't had anything like that," she said later. "I couldn't eat any of it," she recalled. "My stomach rebelled at that kind of food." (A very different scenario from the one Lillian described in a letter to Aloo sent a few weeks later, in which she claimed she and her family had celebrated her homecoming with chocolate cake.) Rosalynn later explained that her mother-in-law told her she couldn't face the food because her stomach had shrunk. This was likely true, Rosalynn wrote, "but we also knew that she felt guilty because her friends in India were still hungry."[36] Perhaps this is why, as Gloria recalled later, "She would only nibble at food but she stored cheese in her refrigerator as if it were precious."[37]

There would be plenty in her first year back home to take Lillian's mind off the troubles of her Indian friends. Her children surprised her with a newly rebuilt Pond House, to replace the older one that had burned down years before. The modern, angular residence was specially designed to maximize light and safeguard her privacy. Built on a rise overlooking the fish pond, ringed by Georgia pines alive with squirrels and birds, the Pond House still offers a quiet that envelopes like a soft blanket, a silence so pure that the flipping of a fish on the pond's still green surface startles like a shot. Through the house's high windows, the pines seem but an extension of life inside the house; the rocky fireplace and chimney are less masonry constructions than natural geological accretions. All is wood and glass, reflections and vistas, but the house's design had practical application, too. Despite all the windows, as Lillian later told a reporter, with characteristic candor, "I can stand in any of the bedrooms and undress and I can sit on the johnny, and nobody can see me from outside."[38] The Carters also installed one of the first satellite dishes for her. "Mama was able to monitor a wide range of televised sporting events," recalled Jimmy Carter, including "the major league achievements of her beloved Dodgers."[39]

Lillian would do far more with her days than sit and read at the Pond House. Over the next ten years, events in which she would play a central part would make her one of the most colorful political personalities in American history. Despite all the glitter that was to come, Lillian Carter never forgot either her Indian or her Peace Corps friends or the problems they had tried to solve. In India she had written, "I can never again take bread or warmth for granted." Nor would she ever be able to live her life without thinking of those who had neither.[40] India had taught her something of significance beyond her own experience: how to translate convictions into actions. "If I had one wish for my children," she wrote in her next to last letter home, "it would be that each of you would dare to do the things and reach for goals in your own lives that have meaning for you as individuals, doing as much as you can for everybody, but not worrying if you don't please everyone." What mattered, she insisted, was that you gave as much as possible, because whatever you gave you received back many times over.[41]

PART III. FIRST MOTHER OF THE WORLD

How could Jimmy ever criticize me? I'm his mama.

—Lillian Carter

CHAPTER 8

Quiet Legend

In 1966, neither the Carters nor Lillian had wished to publicize her Peace Corps tour. Jimmy had been making his first run for governor, and as a family member explained later, "Georgia was generally against the Peace Corps. And Mother didn't want to hurt Jimmy's chances. So she sort of sneaked out of town."[1]

Two years later, it was a very different picture. Lillian didn't have to sneak around anymore—in fact, she did the very opposite. Soon after she arrived home, she began to accept invitations to speak to groups about her experiences in India, about the importance of service and of never allowing age to be a barrier to living a life of giving. Lillian went to these engagements without any text prepared beforehand. She could extemporize for an hour or more, often kicking off her shoes and standing barefoot at the podium. Not surprisingly, she often shocked the more prim members of church congregations with bluntness of language or of information. "Mama was completely unrestrained," remembered Jimmy, especially when discussing the facts of life which were central to why she had been sent to India in the first place. Part of Lillian's immediate charm was that she was a woman who looked like everyone's grandmother. But this grandmother smoked, enjoyed a highball of an evening, played poker, and believed in women leading their own lives, working at jobs and being independent, and never letting their own lives die along with a spouse, like Indian widows performing suttee on a husband's funeral pyre. So when it came time for Jimmy to announce another run at the governor's office, Lillian was happy to walk her talk. From speeches about India and getting the retired out of their chairs and into productive lives of purpose, it was an easy segue into the high politics that for Lillian Carter were just another contact sport. Joining forces with her daughter-in-law Rosalynn made for a dynamic and effective campaign team.[2]

Rosalynn had come a long way since her days as a protected Navy wife. "I'm more political than Jimmy," she would declare of herself; indeed, this was a trait she particularly shared with her mother-in-law.[3] Under her graceful exterior, Rosalynn was hardheaded, focused and shrewd; while softly asking questions she was constantly filing away crucial information she knew would be useful to the campaign, which she wanted to win as much as Jimmy did. She and Lillian journeyed to virtually every county in Georgia, meeting people in a broad variety of places and situations. They visited clubs, churches, school halls, as well as fire houses, and risked getting thrown out over and over again by local K-Marts, which forbade solicitation on their premises. "I went to sea in a shrimp boat," Rosalynn wrote, "and up in a hot-air balloon. I saw my first tobacco auction and even witnessed a rattlesnake roundup." If there were differences between Lillian and Rosalynn, campaigning for a common cause and for a man they both loved allowed them to find and strengthen what they shared and better understand what they didn't. Both women were resilient and compassionate, and they enjoyed the comedy of the human condition rather more than Jimmy, who had earned an undeserved reputation for being restrained to the point of humorlessness.[4]

Lillian tried to loosen up Jimmy's outward stiffness on one very public occasion when she asked him to accompany her to a wrestling match in Columbus, where she was a regular attendee. She probably had to twist his arm, because not many members of her family were willing to sit for long beside her while she cheered, hollered and waved her arms over a sport of which none of them was a fan. Jan Williams, a family friend who would serve as Lillian's correspondence secretary and Amy's schoolteacher before the White House years, often went along with her. Williams thinks Lillian was as happy to attract attention to herself as she was to bestow it on her heroes in the ring. "I think Miss Lillian really knew what she was watching wasn't real," she allows. "She just got so involved and she loved the attention."[5]

Attention was what she had come for that evening. When the emcee introduced Jimmy in his sedate suit and tie as a candidate for governor of Georgia, the room echoed with boos—the last thing this crowd wanted to see holding up the business of wrestling was a politician, even if he was running for highest office in the state. But when they were told that "Jimmy Who?" was the son of Miss Lillian, everyone roared with an applause that was probably as much for her as for him.

A masked man known as Mr. Wrestling II was performing that evening. One of the strongest of the men and holder of numerous championships, Mr. Wrestling II, then in his thirties, was actually named John Walker. His powerful build, effortless strength, and Lillian's faith in the good looks hidden under the balaclava he wore made Walker her all-time favorite. "She came to all my matches in Columbus," Walker says. "She made a point of doing so. There was one time she even came into the dressing room! Fortunately everybody was decent. And I had my mask on, of course."[6]

Lillian introduced Jimmy to Walker, and as Jimmy remembers it, "Mama suggested that we have a photograph made of me subduing [Mr. Wrestling II] with a head lock." Walker recalls suggesting the photo session himself. "I said, 'How about a picture?,' and [Jimmy] said, 'Well, OK,'" he recalls. Walker didn't mean a side by side, arms around the shoulders shot. "'No, throw a headlock on me,'" Walker urged Carter. "So he did! I was then going to pick him up, but thought, hmmm ... maybe I'd better not."[7] A shot of that move, had it occurred, would be of great interest to posterity. However, this photo of the shirt and tie politician with a muscled wrestler under his arm (who was grinning through his mask as if to say, "Yes, I could floor him if I wanted to") became a popular staple of the Carter campaign and reappeared later in books by and about Carter. The photo op no doubt delighted Lillian, but it also served a canny strategy. If everyone believed that what they saw in the ring was real, Lillian was not one to spoil their theater. She knew that politics and sporting events had much in common— that in order to participate fully in politics, as in professional wrestling, one had to suspend reality, as one did at a theatrical performance, and root for one's hero till he won the contest. She wanted Jimmy to adopt some of the same techniques that made professional wrestling such successful theatre. The politics of her day, which were those of Jim Jack Gordy, couldn't afford to dwell so subjectively in a fortress of personal faith. As she once complained to a reporter, she wished Jimmy would "quit that stuff about never telling a lie and being a Christian."[8] Those older politics demanded donning of masks and assuming of roles to suit a particular audience, and the willingness to coast on the small lies that are the trump cards of a nimble and flexible politician. There was not the luxury of always being in a position to tell the truth, a fact of politics that Jimmy was to accept more during this campaign than in any before or after. He would court conservatives whose votes he needed as much as those of progressives. Black as well as white voters would distrust Carter for what his Democratic and Republic rivals were to accuse him of in the presidential race—of being two-faced, of turning whichever way the wind blew, and at first this was believed to have cost him a substantial portion of the black vote. But in politics, as Jim Jack Gordy well knew and as his grandson was divining, sometimes you had to shake hands with the devil. And no other image of Carter in a campaign described his situation so powerfully as this photograph with Mr. Wrestling II, when Jimmy found himself out-endorsed, out-spent, and almost out-won by Republican "Cufflinks Carl" Sanders. Yet the Carter team had what Jimmy called "a last minute surge," which included black votes that the Democratic primary results had not encouraged him to rely on. It was enough, and more than enough, to put the well-funded Sanders campaign into a headlock and win the election "handily." Lillian might well have said, "It's all in the mask, honey."[9]

On the night of the balls celebrating Jimmy Carter's inauguration as seventy-sixth governor of Georgia, a cavalcade of limousines made its way through the dark, wet winter streets of Atlanta. After Jimmy and Rosalynn's came the car carrying Lillian and her younger sister Emily Dolvin. With them were Emily's husband, Bill Dolvin, whom Lillian had co-opted as her escort for the evening. A state trooper detailed to be Emily's escort completed the quartet.

Having spent her younger years as a member of the extended Carter family in Archery, Emily had helped Lillian and Earl around the farm, and had watched the Carter children grow up. She then went to college to become a teacher. She married William Dolvin, a school principal, had children of her own, and in their hometown of Roswell, a suburb north of Atlanta, they became prominent in civic and cultural affairs. So close was Jimmy to the Dolvins that their home in Roswell, next door to Bulloch Hall, home of the mother of President Theodore Roosevelt, was known as the "Roswell White House." A charming personality and a careful manager, Emily was capable of seducing whole groups of people to the cause and then getting them to do whatever needed doing, which was usually a great deal. All of this was why Jimmy had summarily put Emily in charge of organizing a post-inauguration reception at the Governor's Mansion, a two story brick residence with porches supported by thirty white columns and rooms filled with carefully selected antiques, paintings and carpets. The doors were opened to anyone who wanted to attend. To handle what were assumed to be around five thousand people, Emily had summoned an army of one hundred and twenty ladies from around the state to serve as hostesses, and was assisted in everything by Lillian. Even Emily's organizational skills were challenged when more than twice the expected number of guests showed up. "When we finally had to break up the receiving line," Emily recalled, "there were still lines going out both doors, both directions, down the street for as far as you could see." Jimmy and Rosalynn had been up since dawn but each took a line and shook the hands of everyone until they were through—all twelve thousand of them. Some of the guests were so enthusiastic, recalled Rosalynn, that her hand was often painfully crushed; one well-wisher came at her so forcefully she almost fell over.[10]

Sitting in their limousine, their faces strobed by the flashing lights of their police escort and the cameras of the press, the Gordy sisters were both weary but happy, buoyed up on the day's adrenaline and the thrill of celebrating Jimmy's victory. Yet as the procession moved along, Lillian suddenly turned to her sister and said, "Sissy. What are we doing here?" Emily commented, "This said a lot to me." Even when interviewed years later, her jumbled recollection betrayed the giddiness she still felt from that inaugural night. "I know that she was thinking the same thing I was: you know, only here in the United States could a thing like this—in Georgia, really, how could a family like ours—for Jimmy to do what he had done—to become Governor, I mean it was just really something!"[11] Whatever her doubts about whether this was the kind of thing that was supposed to happen to her "kind of family," on the day of Jimmy's swearing in Lillian was radiant and regal in a pale tailored dress and jacket, and had reason to hold her head a little higher when, partway through his inaugural address, Jimmy offered words that seemed heavy to speak but exhilarating to say: that "the time for racial discrimination is over." This simple statement, which his mother had put into action every day of his life, more than any of the other ideals he voiced that morning, delighted and dismayed people not just in Atlanta but across the country. Editors took notice; soon, articles were being published about a "New South," and Jimmy made the cover of the May 31, 1971, *Time* Magazine, a banner above his head reading "Dixie Whistles a Different Tune." Suddenly, a part of the nation which for many Americans symbolized racism, bigotry, and entrenched poverty was seen turning a fresh and much younger face toward the light than any previous cadre of southern politicians had ever done before. Governor Carter would live up to this press, taking as swift a broom to race-based hiring practices of the former regime as he did to the underbrush which had accumulated in every department of state government. During this time of upheaval and change, both his wife and mother did as governors' wives and mothers had done in years past, presiding over the mansion's hospitality needs. When Rosalynn was not available to give tours of the mansion, Lillian would do so in her characteristic down-to-earth style. However, Governor Carter found more important things to do with Rosalynn's and Lillian's time and talents than explain antique furniture to tourists, however much they and the public enjoyed this. As a member of the Governor's Commission to Improve Services for the Mentally and Emotionally Handicapped, Rosalynn was instrumental in shepherding the Commission's recommendations through to law, laying the groundwork for her greater involvement in mental health issues during and after the White House years. And because of her medical and social services background, Lillian was appointed to the Board of Governors of the Department of Human Resources. Sitting on a board was not Lillian Carter's idea of how best to spend her time, and it wasn't on the Board of Governors that she did much of importance. Out in the field, however, was another matter. Tasked with visiting all the agencies and institutions the Department was responsible for and reporting back any concerns or needs, Lillian worked hard at this aspect of her job, sending Jimmy reports written in professional style and, when required, badgered him as only a governor's mother had leave to do. Lillian needed to be needed, and though this work was more bureaucratic than the hands-on experiences she had had in Vikhroli, it was fulfilling in that it allowed her to visit hospitals, welfare offices, homes for the elderly, and generally places where people went for help. Her reports often included such specific requests it was clear she had made time to talk not just with administrators but with individuals receiving services, the rank and file that had always attracted her. Her hands-on efforts brought a deluge of calls and letters, which she forwarded to Jimmy with nudging little notes, insisting his full attention be given to each case.[12]

This was what Lillian had been preparing for since walking into the office of the rich Mr. Godrej in 1967 and asking him to do the right thing, the humane and compassionate thing, whatever the cost in money or trouble. It was a technique she would continue to use—leaning on those with much, whether a President of the United States or a private tycoon, to benefit those with nothing.

Kim Carter Fuller has vivid memories of when her grandmother took her to Hawaii in 1973.

It was Jimmy Carter's second year as governor. "Grandmama always gave us trips when we graduated from high school," she says. "She took me to Hawaii—because she wanted to go, too, of course! We set off for what was to be a two week vacation. We stayed a week on Oahu, then we moved on to Kauai. That evening we went to a restaurant and were waiting in an area downstairs. Grandmama got mad because some people had come in after us but had been seated. So she said, 'I'm going upstairs!'" Not for the first or the last time, Lillian's temper got the better of her. "She walked up the stairs, and I'll never forget it—she fell from the top of the stairs down to the bottom," recalls Fuller. "Luckily there was a waiter behind her. But she broke her shoulder, and at her age they would not set it." Kim, a sixteen year old who had never been this far away from home, had to take over. It was the middle of the night in Atlanta and the switchboard at the Governor's Mansion wouldn't take her call. She finally reached a State Patrolman named Stock Coleman who got her through to Jimmy. "For two days," she says, "Grandmama was in bed with her shoulder strapped. I was scared to death!" Then came another fright: as they were getting on the plane to go home, with Fuller pushing Lillian's wheelchair, they found that "my name wasn't included on the list," Fuller laughs. "I was stranded in Hawaii! Grandmama told me not to worry, that it would be OK." Despite having no ticket, Kim did get on the plane. They were flying somewhere between Texas and Georgia when Lillian announced to her granddaughter, "You're going to have to change my clothes. I'm not getting off this plane dirty." In the plane's restroom, somehow Kim managed to bathe her grandmother and dress her in a fresh set of clothes. "And then she said, 'Do not cry when you see your mama.' When we got to Atlanta and she was being taken in to the hospital, Grandmama pulled me aside and asked, 'Did you cry?' I said, 'No, ma'am.' She said, 'You cried, I know you did!' She taught me so much about being independent, about being ready to handle anything." Had she only known it, Lillian was going to need to be ready for anything herself.[13]

It was while she and her shoulder were still recovering in her bedroom at the Governor's Mansion one night in 1973 that Jimmy came in and sat down on the edge of her bed, thunked his feet on a coffee table, and announced that he was going to run for president. After ordering him to put his feet back on the floor, Lillian made a remark that has passed into classic Miss Lillian lore. "President of what?" she asked drily.[14]

In April, three months into the 1976 Democratic primaries, Lillian told the story a bit differently to reporter Walt Smith. In her version, it was *she* who initiated the conversation about Jimmy's post-gubernatorial prospects. "What are you going to do," she asked Jimmy, "when you're not governor anymore?" Jimmy answered, "I'll run for president." "It shocked me," Lillian told Smith, "but after five minutes I realized he was in earnest." Her first worry, Lillian said, before Jimmy's or her family's safety, or indeed what might happen to her family should Jimmy be elected, was where the money for the campaign was to come from.[15] If the Carters were short on campaign cash, they had no shortage of human resources. The campaign of 1976 was nominally won by Jimmy Carter's charisma and his sunny promises of better times to come, but his family and his supporters won the election alongside him. Jimmy, Rosalynn, their sons and daughters-in-law, Aunt Emily Dolvin, and many friends from Plains and elsewhere formed what came to be called the Peanut Brigade. They fanned out across the country with message and strategy almost military in precision and thoroughness. Emily started by volunteering in the Atlanta campaign office, then went to Maine, where she became something of a one woman tactical unit, winning that state over to Jimmy Carter as much with her charm as with the Carter campaign promises. This was only half the battle in a climate most of the Brigade campaigners had never experienced to this extent before. Besides the cold, they had to contend with a certain prejudice from some Northerners. Rick Hutto was part of the team that went to New Hampshire, and recalls that the difficulty was not only convincing people to vote for Carter but to take his campaigners seriously. "For some reason, people in the north saw us all as unlettered hicks," he remembers. "One man answered the door. I said, 'Hi, I'm Rick Hutto. I'm campaigning here for Jimmy Carter.' He said, 'May I ask you a question?,' and I thought, oh good, because I had studied all of the issues and knew exactly what answers to give. He said, 'Where are you from originally?' I said, 'I'm a ninth generation Georgian.' He said, 'Where did you go away to school?' I answered, 'My degree is from the University of Georgia.' And he said, 'But you talk so intelligently!'" This was a time, Hutto points out, "when nobody thought Jimmy Carter had any hope at all. I remember thinking, if nothing else, maybe this campaign will change the way Southerners are viewed." As it happened, Carter won the New Hampshire primary, which moved the press to dub him the official Democratic front-runner. It was soon clear even to naysayers that Carter and his people were anything but ignorant hayseeds.[16]

While the Peanut Brigade strove mightily in the north, Lillian declared that she would be most useful to the cause by staying home in Plains to take care of nine year old Amy. Yet as Ray Hathcock, the Georgia State Patrolman who served as combination bodyguard/personal assistant to Lillian, pointed out, even in this supposed retirement, "She always managed to arrange to be the star of the show."[17]

The decommissioned Seaboard Coast Line station in the middle of Plains had been transformed into Carter campaign headquarters. Freshly whitewashed and spiffed up with flowers and furniture, including rocking chairs that became so indelible a part of the building that they are still there, the station served as the epicenter of the campaign and also the eye of a sudden storm of commercial attention. Plastered with posters and campaign materials (also still there), the little depot reflected what was happening to Plains. Virtually overnight, every shop along the street bristled and flapped with the cheap and gaudy objects that are the camp followers of all political campaigns—from pictures, posters, stickers, pencils, to the higher grade memorabilia like golden peanut pins and packets of real peanuts (and everything conceivable that could be made from them). Campaign buttons popped up like weeds, including one showing Lillian gazing at Jimmy with tender amusement. Around them both was the encircling slogan, "Senior Citizens Count On Jimmy Carter," as if to say that if a mother like Lillian could count on a son like Jimmy, America's senior citizens could count on him also. At the center of all this chaos was the smiling doyenne of Plains, Miss Lillian, sitting in a rocking chair either on the platform or inside the depot, where tourists lined up for hours to see but not touch her (unless, of course, they were young and good-looking men). "She loved for people to get her autograph," recalls Jan Williams, "or to talk about her son who was running for president, or about Amy," though on one memorable occasion she was seen to react with barely concealed displeasure when a squalling infant was thrust in her face.[18]

Lillian's integral importance to the campaign, not just as a cipher to appeal to seniors, appears in one of the first television commercials of Carter's campaign. Jimmy and Rosalynn are seen riding triumphantly into a train station and waving to cheering crowds from the caboose of their train. The scene cuts to black and white photographs chronicling Jimmy's Depression-era childhood, then back to the present with Jimmy in plaid shirt and jeans at the edge of a field, talking about how hard he had worked as a child and how this ethic became the foundation of his political platform. Then we cut suddenly to Lillian. She's asked by an off camera interviewer what Jimmy was like as a child and whether she had ever spanked him. This was a theme running alongside the idealized image of Jimmy as an almost incredibly well-behaved boy, which Lillian in her outspokenness was always in danger of overturning. For the campaign commercial, Lillian flatly denies ever spanking Jimmy, only to react to prompting like an actress who's been reminded she has spoken the wrong lines (in this case the prompter is Jimmy). "All right," Lillian admits to the camera, with a southern belle tilt of the head, "maybe I gave him a little lick now and then, in passing."[19]

The Carter campaign had figured out that any time Lillian opened her mouth to a crowd or on television, she offered two images key to gaining the vote: that the strictness and honesty of Carter's upbringing had molded the moral and trustworthy man he promised to be as president, and that the candidate's mother was as liberal in her social beliefs as she was in her maternal responsibilities, but that like any other liberal, or mother, she had her human side, too. Perhaps there was a third message: that thanks to such a mother, Jimmy Carter also had a refreshingly human side. Lillian once said, "I don't know how Jimmy can be completely honest and still be successful in politics," and she got away with it because everyone knew she was speaking a universal truth applicable to all politicians.[20] "Miss Lillian had always been a woman ahead of her time," remembers Jan Williams. "She could play poker with the best, she could drink with the best, she could cuss better than some men, though it kind of flowed when *she* did it! It was something you had to accept about her, because it was all part of who she was." When she was interviewed in Plains, a few weeks before the 1976 election, just after the furor over Jimmy Carter's interview in Playboy Magazine had washed across the country, Lillian co-opted the opinions of the clergy to bolster her own positive opinion of the interview. For about two minutes, she told reporters, she was "stunned," but after receiving some ten telephone calls from ministers from across America, who told her they were in favor of the interview, Lillian decided she loved it, too, and that "it was a plus instead of a minus." This was a "Rose Kennedy without the hair dye" and a broadly vernacular vocabulary, fiercely loyal to her son yet not afraid of telling him what she thought was wrong with his decisions, who faced her audience and said what she thought, intent on making her opinions count for something. At some point during the campaign, Lillian's adherence to what was real to her moved people to see Jimmy's candidacy in light of her candid, unvarnished truthfulness. The Carter campaign could have filmed a hundred more commercials showing their flannel and denim candidate making promises in a peanut field. But without Lillian to counterbalance the ideal with the down-to-earth, a large segment of Jimmy Carter's popularity might never have materialized as it did.[21]

Australian journalist Lenore Nicklin visited the Plains depot in June 1976 and cheerfully pronounced it "the most delightful campaign premises I will probably ever see." Since the depot was the domain of Miss Lillian, Nicklin wasn't surprised when just as she arrived Lillian drove up in her blue Caprice Classic. But if she expected Lillian to behave like other grandmothers, she got a rude awakening. In a similar vein, Walter Cronkite would innocently ask Lillian why it was that Americans loved her so much. Lillian tilted her head coyly and replied with an acid smile, "It's because I'm so *sweet*!"—"sweet" having a decidedly negative connotation in Lillian Carter's dictionary. When the unsuspecting Nicklin asked Lillian about Jimmy's chances in the election, Lillian barked at her, "Everybody knows he's a damn nice man. Everybody knows he's brilliant. Everybody knows he'll make a damn fine President." "If much of the South seems as sweet and syrupy as a mint julep," Nicklin concluded, "Miss Lillian comes across as a dry Hunter [Valley] red ... tough, shrewd and humorous."[22]

When asked if she was prepared for the goldfish bowl existence of being a president's wife, Rosalynn once pointed out that as she had always lived in a village of some six hundred people who knew everybody else's business, it would be no great challenge to find herself the object of scrutiny. Lillian, on the other hand, had never endured Plains' attention—namely that of its female contingent—willingly. Which is likely one of the reasons why she didn't care for women journalists. She was convinced, she told Robert Scheer, that if what she told a woman reporter wasn't of sufficient interest, "they touch it up a bit.... I'm just kind of suspicious of a woman writer until I know where I stand."[23] If they were pushy and professional, she would cut them short; if they were accommodating and polite, she suspected they were having her on. When the professional *and* gracious Georgie Anne Geyer of the *Los Angeles Times* came to interview her in spring 1976, Lillian said as much in print. "I hope you are not so sweet," she warned Geyer. "All the women journalists come here and, by the time they've complimented me so much, I don't trust them at all."[24] Jody Powell, Carter's Press Secretary, once requested that Lillian meet with a special reporter from *The Washington Post*, but when he told Lillian the reporter was a woman she said the deal was off. Jimmy helped convince her to sit for the interview. Unfortunately, the reporter made the mistake of pressing Lillian about whether Jimmy had really never told a lie. She finally admitted that Jimmy may have told a little white lie now and then. What, pressed the woman, was *her* definition of a white lie? "Well do you remember a few minutes ago when I met you at the door," Lillian replied, "and said that you look very nice and that I was glad to see you?"[25]

On the other hand, Lillian tended to offer male journalists a very different reception. "Men impress me," she once said. "I love 'em. I love 'em more than women."[26] To Walt Smith, whom she invited to the Pond House, she confessed that despite her strong belief that Jimmy would be elected president, it had taken her a while to come to grips with his decision to run. This was a startling about-face to all her assurances that Jimmy had the election in the palm of his hand. "It was just too big a thing for me to take in," she told Smith. "I'm scared to say it," she added, with the touch of vulnerability she normally confined to her letters. "But he says he's going to win and I think he will." Underscoring the fact that first and foremost she was a grandmother, Lillian pointed out how happy she was to be at home in Plains caring for Amy while the family was out on the road. Amy kept her young, she said. Few female reporters ever found her this accommodating.[27]

Shortly before Lenore Nicklin's visit, African American journalist Orde Coombs arrived in Plains on assignment from *New York Magazine*, and he was as wary of Lillian as he was of her son. Carter was the most successful politician of the year, Coombs wrote, and perhaps that was possible because he was "a man who is so Janus-faced, they say, that he is able to win the fervor of disparate people who ought to be natural antagonists," which echoed the criticisms of Jerry Brown, Frank Church and other candidates. Coombs trusted Carter's mother even less—hers, after all, was the hand that had rocked his cradle. How concerned had she really been about civil rights? What had this well-to-do white southern woman ever done to help black people? he wondered. Coombs shared his misgivings with an elderly black lady he knew. Aunt Bessie lived in New York but had been born in Georgia. Though a devout Republican, Bessie set Coombs straight on the matter of principle. It was *because* of Lillian Carter, she said, that she planned to cast her first Democratic vote—for Jimmy Carter. "You young people don't know nothing, do you?" she said. "You don't know that there are quality white people," she added, "even though most of them are non-quality." Lillian Carter, she explained, had nursed blacks in Georgia when no white person would have anything to do with them, and that was good enough for Aunt Bessie. Then Coombs checked out the story with Andrew J. Young. Young had first met Lillian at a meeting of the Georgia Educational Association in 1970, the only non-black woman in the group. Young heard her talking about how her father prized his friendship with Bishop Johnson, reading the Bible and singing hymns on the front porch, and how she and her father admired the shiny Packard the bishop drove and appreciated his success. "This said to me that this woman as a child learned to look up to black people," Young recalls. "We hit it off almost immediately"—and indeed, Lillian was a refreshing revelation to Young, coming from Sumter County, infamous as the place where black activists had been harassed and jailed and black churches burned. Lillian told Young that as she had delivered all the black babies in Sumter County, she considered all of them *her* children, and wouldn't let Earl's (or the townspeople's) disapproval stop her from inviting them to the house for a chat. "I realized that she and the Koinonia Farms people were probably the only ones who would not toe the line on race," Young says. "This was an exceptionally strong woman." On another occasion, Young asked her why she seldom went to church. "Well, this is her story," he remembers: "that she would sit on the front porch and as all the hypocrites would go to church she would sit there sipping Jack Daniels from a teacup. She didn't want them to think it was tea, so she always left the bottle right out on the table. I admired that spirit," as he did the compassion and courage that led her to volunteer with the Peace Corps. When Young assured Coombs that Lillian was indeed "one of the truly great women of our time," Coombs decided then that he had to meet this "quiet legend."[28]

Still, Coombs didn't venture to Plains entirely convinced. He showed up on Lillian's doorstep, with photographer Betsy Karel, and out she came to meet them, wearing a pale blue pantsuit and blue canvas shoes and flashing the "Carter smile." Shaking Coombs' hand, she drew him "into the vortex of her 'Southern charm,'" he recorded, by noting with many fussy asides that insects were chewing up her entire lawn, that she'd never seen the like, and that he must come in but do mind the step, it had tripped ever so many newsmen before him, though they all pretended they hadn't seen it, and where did he want to sit, and wasn't the sun too much for him over there. It was indeed that "vortex" of pleasantly (and sometimes irritatingly) distracting chatter known to anybody who has ever visited a southern grandmother. Coombs refused to be taken in at first, though he did help Lillian adjust her chair and made small talk about her favorite soap operas, which she was delighted to expound on. He agreed that she was tailor made for the optics of a political campaign.[29]

Before he could poke holes in that image, Lillian distracted him again, this time by sharing one of her confessions. She admitted to Coombs that she had never had any close friends, that she often found herself isolated by her belief system among people who did not understand her. Coombs refused to take the bait. Why should anyone cast their vote for her son? he asked. Because Jimmy Carter was hardworking, she replied, he was intelligent, and he was utterly devoted to his country. "And his heart is full of love and compassion," she added. Coombs would not be seduced. The same could be said for the man who ran his local delicatessen in New York City, Coombs replied. He was a nice guy, but he wouldn't want to see him as President of the United States. Lillian agreed, but then what her son was doing had little in common with selling cold cuts. The former nurse who could always detect who in a crowd was sicker than anyone else seemed to see in Coombs the latent anger that she touched on next. Lillian told him it seemed to her that there were a lot of angry young black people whose resentments barred them from recognizing and appreciating the efforts of those whites who were trying to begin to heal the wounds of slavery and Jim Crow. Older black people knew exactly how bad things used to be, she pointed out. She was plenty well old enough to tell him just how blacks were treated in the Deep South before the war, before Rosa Parks and Dr. King—the sitting at the back of buses, the restrictions on where blacks could eat, have a drink of water, use the restroom, in a part of the country so laced with the mines of prejudice a special booklet was often carried by northern blacks visiting the south, so they would know which trouble spots to avoid. For the most part, Lillian said, people Coombs' age hadn't experienced what their parents and grandparents had endured; they had not suffered directly from these experiences, but felt whites needed to pay for them. Not, she added, that blacks were not justified in this, citing the racism she still saw, for example, in the elder generation of the Carter family.[30]

Indeed the race question was one that often got Lillian herself into heated discussions, because she disliked outsiders' oversimplified interpretations of what black and white relations were about in southern communities. When Robert Scheer asked Lillian in the mid–1970s about her family's relationship with Koinonia Farms, the biracial community outside Plains that had suffered so much abuse from local bigotry from the 1940s till the 1960s, he was taken aback "by a rare flash of anger." Why did he want to bring that up? she demanded. "It's all over with. You'd just stir up some of the wilder people around here, and then nobody knows what will happen." What may have frustrated Lillian and people like her—people who were living within the situations that to the outside world seemed as easily summarized as the plot of a novel—was that she had spent all her life in a world of unratified but no less real social contracts between black and white, white and black; in which what seemed to the outside world a parable of white oppressing black was far different when viewed from within. Coombs saw that from a distance, the story of the Carters, of Plains, of the race issue, was literally black and white, and distorted. When you got closer to it, you saw the complexities, the ironies, and especially how being a southern hero in the civil rights movement was not as easy as it sounded.[31]

Lillian later drove Coombs to her pond, where she allowed herself to be photographed with rod and reel. Despite Coombs' best efforts to keep her to topics related to Jimmy's fitness for the White House, she just shared more of her heart—her love of the squirrels that scrambled up and down the tall pines, how wonderful the breeze felt against her outstretched arms, how happy she was to be alone with these untroubling things. "We are all in communion with God," she gently corrected Coombs when he asked her if it bothered her, too, to hear Jimmy talk as if he had a hotline to Heaven. Did she pray for Jimmy to win, Coombs wanted to know. Lillian replied she did not, with a finality that announced that after this answer, the subject of prayer and religion was at an end. "Just that all will be right for him," she said. By the end of the interview, Coombs had to agree that Jimmy Carter's mother was a dreamer like her son, but one who had actually worked to make large dreams into reality. Dreaming with tangible results, Coombs wrote, was a weakness in Carter's seemingly impenetrable defenses. It was the reason "why he plays it both ways. For he was born to a land that boasts only of pine trees, peanuts and corn.... It is a land from which all dreamers must flee or go mad." Plains was Lillian's world, too, and dreaming had always been her strength, even as it had so often sent her away to far places in search of who she really was. Jimmy Carter, Coombs concluded, was not doing anything his mother hadn't already done herself. Whether he was capable of out-dreaming her remained to be seen.[32]

CHAPTER 9

First Mother

When a reporter from the *Palm Beach Daily* arrived in Plains on the evening of the 1976 presidential election, the business block and the train depot were lit up by floodlights somebody had put on top of the water tower. The *Daily*'s Judith Clemence found people crowded anxiously around the depot, and the town itself eerily like a movie set, shivery with anticipation. "The ambience was much the same," she wrote, "the scurrying about before the director calls for action, the awed silence that follows." Billy Carter's son Buddy remembered all this and something else, a sort of tidal wave of sound. There were "bands playing and speakers speaking," he wrote, "and the noise rolled from the streets of the town all the way to the peanut fields and pine forests on the outskirts."[1] Ironically, the main draw, Jimmy and Rosalynn, were not there. They were staying in an Atlanta hotel to watch the returns come in and, everyone on the Carter team hoped and prayed, to preside over the victory party.

People might have expected Lillian to be in Atlanta, too. After all, she had been a prominent presence before and during the Democratic Convention in New York City that July. In a social round that was to be echoed throughout the Carter years, over a few days Lillian met Katherine Graham and Ben Bradlee of the *Washington Post* (when Graham introduced Lillian to Barbara Walters, the latter asked for an interview and got the same brush off as any other woman journalist received before and after); Walter Cronkite asked her to sit in his box the night of the convention, causing what Lillian called "a little controversy"; Shirley MacLaine invited her to her show at the Palace and on admiring Lillian's peanut-adorned pocketbook in the dressing room afterward, was given it as a present; and Tom

Snyder interviewed her for *Tomorrow*, almost causing another "controversy." When Lillian turned on her television at 3 a.m. the morning of the convention, she watched as Tom Hayden, another guest of Snyder's, asked a million viewers, "How can Jimmy Carter lose when he has Miss Lillian? Miss Lillian with her lovely ideas about civil rights and her liberal ideas which we have been fighting for all these years." Lillian admitted she was afraid Jimmy would disapprove.[2]

Jimmy later recalled how vocal his mother was regarding appointments she thought he should make once he was elected president, and how especially impressed she was by Texan Barbara Jordan, the first African American woman to be elected to the House of Representatives. Jordan's keynote speech, quoting from Thomas Jefferson and from Abraham Lincoln and stressing the need for community across all perceived boundaries, riveted Lillian, and she put Jimmy on notice that she wanted him to consider Jordan for an important post in his administration. However, it wasn't the next highest office she had in mind. "My choice for vice president is Wendell Anderson," Lillian explained. Was she especially impressed by the Minnesota governor's intellect, or political judgment, or that he had made the cover of *Time* Magazine three years earlier, posing with a fish he presumably caught himself (another brownie point in Lillian's book)? Actually, no. "It's because he's so good-looking," Lillian admitted, "and he speaks so-o-o-o beautifully." (So much for the women's movement when a handsome and well spoken man was around.)[3]

Columbus *Enquirer-Ledger* reporter Richard Hyatt was present for most of Jimmy Carter's meetings with vice presidential candidates, most of whom were asked to come to Plains. "I remember when Jimmy took John Glenn out to a peanut field," he says, "and the time Ed Muskie walked back to town from Jimmy and Rosalynn's house wearing blue jeans with a sports shirt and dress shoes." Neither man looked as if he belonged there. Walter Mondale, however, was just what Lillian ordered. "When Mondale came to town, Miss Lillian acted like a kid at a rock concert," recalls Hyatt. "She said, 'He's *pretty*!'" The Mondales were put up at the Pond House, where Lillian met them at the door and showed them around the house. "She then took Mondale into the kitchen and said, as if revealing a huge secret, that under the sink she kept something he might like," says Hyatt. "It was her bourbon."[4]

On the evening of July 15, 1976, Rosalynn had sat with Muriel Humphrey and other friends and family in crowded Madison Square Garden, a forest of brightly colored placards waving at her feet. Jimmy, according to custom, was elsewhere—he was, in fact, with Lillian in his hotel room, along with Amy and grandson Jason, and a horde of reporters and photographers. When Ohio brought in the delegates needed for Carter to reach the necessary 1505, the arena erupted in cheers. The press then descended on Rosalynn, who suddenly felt both unprotected and lonely for her husband. "I knew he was celebrating with Miss Lillian," Rosalynn wrote later, "and I wanted to be there too." When a television journalist sat down beside her and asked what message she had for her husband, all she could think of to say was, "Tell him we won!," as if he were thousands of miles rather than a few blocks away.[5] The reporters in Jimmy's hotel suite captured a very different image, one of family intimacy, with mother and son seated on the sofa watching the television, their hands clasped. But Lillian knew how much Jimmy wanted to be with his wife. "Jimmy said, 'Oh, I'd just give anything in the world to be over there,'" she recalled. When Rosalynn came on the television screen and said, "Oh, I wish he was here," Lillian told an interviewer, "Tears rolled down his cheeks."[6]

Back home in Plains again, Lillian was at the center of the action. A month before election day, and just after Jimmy's fifty-second birthday, Lillian had presided over what came to be called the "Million Dollar Supper." For this fundraiser held at her sanctuary, the Pond House, over four hundred guests—ranging from local and state supporters to Cornelius Vanderbilt Whitney and wife Marylou and National Democratic Committee Chairman Robert Strauss—arrived to walk up the pine-needled driveway to the house where, for $5,000 a plate, they sampled from a menu that touched on every delicacy of Deep South cooking. As Secret Service agents loitered around the barbecue pit and the pine-studded outskirts of the grounds, hams, chickens, turkeys, salads, casseroles, puddings, pies and gallons of sweet tea were refreshed from the kitchen by ladies of the Peanut Brigade, and at 5 p.m. sharp Lillian herself arrived, wearing a white pants suit and white shoes. With her white hair, the clothes made it easy to spot her diminutive figure in the increasingly darkening evening as she made the rounds, graceful chatelaine and shrewd political operator. "Honey, I am so glad you could come," she said to each of the hostesses.[7] By the evening's end, well over a million dollars had been raised for the Carter campaign.

Then she hit the campaign trail herself.

Though Lillian had declared it her intention to stay in Plains and look after Amy, the lure of politics beckoned, as did the fact that Jimmy Carter's team knew his mother was one of the best public relations weapons any candidate had had for generations. With Richard Harden, Carter's campaign finance manager who would be named Director of the White

House Office of Administration and Special Assistant for Information Management, Lillian flew to events in Connecticut and New York City, and the response she received was so positive it was clear to everyone on the campaign that they needed to make the best possible use of her popularity. As Harden recalls, "We hadn't realized till then just how much Miss Lillian could influence people to vote for Jimmy. They saw her qualities and figured Jimmy's were the same, which they were." So after some rapid scheduling, Lillian boarded a Lear jet with Harden and made twenty-one campaign stops in the Midwest between Wednesday, October 27 and election day. "We'd get into a town and spend the night, then do an event in the morning," he remembers, "and go to another place for an event in the evening, and another couple of places next day. She kept up the pace really well. And she was fun to be with."[8]

So it would have been the logical culmination of the election cycle for Lillian to show up beside her son and daughter-in-law in Atlanta, to bask in the glow of Jimmy's coming triumph and the spotlight of her own celebrity, which had increased exponentially with each television or newspaper interview or public appearance. But Lillian opted to stay out of the way. Plains was scarcely a quieter choice than Atlanta; she spent election day holding court at the depot, surrounded by fans and cameras and bedlam. Maybe she was again serving a strategic purpose, keeping to her post in the obscure little town now known throughout the world. Maybe she was instructed to keep the lights on in Plains while history was being made in Atlanta. But perhaps there is a simpler reason for why Lillian stayed behind. Billy had decided to stay behind, too.

We might easily conjecture why Billy was not present for his brother's moment of glory. Jimmy's return after Earl's death had destroyed Billy's dream of taking over the family's business interests, but there was plenty else to set two brothers against each other. If Jimmy's exemplary life appeared to run in straight-edge fashion, Billy's would always zigzag, thrown off by an unanticipated and long resented detour that would ultimately take him off the rails completely. Billy's son Buddy remembered hearing about a locally famous fight his father and uncle were said to have had under the Plains water tower. "I can only imagine most of what went on that day," Buddy wrote, "because even those who witnessed it are still, forty-odd years later, strangely reluctant to talk about it." His mother Sybil would only say that it had been brewing since Jimmy's return. Billy, said Sybil in a memoir co-written with her husband, was upset that Lillian had not held on to the family business until the time was right for him to take charge of it. "The problem," Sybil added, "is that he was lost and hurt, and he didn't know how to express it." Buddy had personally witnessed his father storm out of the warehouse on several occasions, shouting over his shoulder that Jimmy was not his boss. Yet Billy always came back. So when Jimmy asked him to run the businesses while he pursued his political career, Billy agreed.[9]

Billy was never a hapless victim of fate. In Jimmy's absence, he had found means to establish himself as a fixture in the town, much as his father had done, though in a completely different manner. He bought an Amoco gas station, a single bay structure with a couple of pumps and a front office with pop machine and candy dispensers. It was located kitty corner and across the tracks from the business block where his father had made his fortune and from the train depot where Jimmy's was also being made. For a time, the gas station would reap tangible rewards for Billy. After his brother was elected, Billy bragged to friends that he had sold over $1 million in gasoline to tourists as gaga over "Billy gas" as they were over his potable liquid, Billy Beer. Gloria Carter Spann would tell a reporter at this time of her concerns for Billy. Friends, she said, were always asking her if Billy was OK. "Has the presidency gone to his head?" they wondered. The answer was "yes"—but in the beginning, Billy's rise as a media celebrity had the aspect of harmless clown comedy. Thanks to the hoopla descending on Plains, the station became as iconic a landmark as the depot and was often a place where the press corps congregated to egg Billy on to greater flights of fancy as beers were opened and inhibitions dispensed with. "The station was home to some of the greatest liars and bullshit artists in the history of the world," recalled Buddy Carter. When the press invaded Plains with their notepads and tape recorders, ever hopeful of a scoop, these locals made "a light snack" out of many a bewildered reporter. "He absolutely *loved* to do the country bumpkin thing with Yankee journalists," recalls Rick Hutto, "who would report that here was this hick sitting in his service station drinking beer and eating peanuts. Yet the moment I'd read that I would discount the rest of the story, because Billy Carter was allergic to peanuts"— despite all the scrutiny, Billy and his compatriots managed to shovel over this one well-kept Carter family secret. Billy was dubbed "a country Don Rickles," but a hick he definitely was not. Ambassador Andrew J. Young once came to see Billy in Plains. "I went in the back of his store," he recalls, "and he had books all over the place. I just started picking up the books that he was reading that I had read, and we basically talked about books. When Miss Lillian said Billy was her smartest child, she was probably telling the truth."[10]

The station and, by extension, Plains, was the one place where being

Billy Carter meant something—where it was okay to be the irreligious, beer-drinking, expletive-happy younger son of a family of super-achievers, where nobody would guess he couldn't eat peanuts or that he studied the philosophy of Søren Kierkegaard. It was a convenient mask for a closet intellectual who would leave at his death a library of thousands of books, who was nothing like the shallow buffoon he eagerly and tragically helped the press create.

Beth Tartan always remembered how on that election night, she went into the kitchen of Billy's and Sybil's home and saw the red wall telephone dangling off the hook. It stayed that way till morning. None of the folks gathered in the living room, where three televisions were "going full blast," wanted to be interrupted by the media or the curious. Buddy Carter was then in his teens, and at first the circus atmosphere revved him like the beers he filched while his mother wasn't looking. Alcohol, Buddy recalled, was flowing in the Carter house like water down a steep hill. On the porch stood kegs of beer; "there were uncountable bottles of liquor" as well, Buddy remembered. He went downtown to check out the mayhem developing there, where some hundred thousand people were making it impossible to move, then came home to find much the same scene. Every room was packed with people he had never seen before, "and they were all drunk," he recalled. Billy had opened the door to anyone and everyone. "In true Billy Carter fashion, he'd gone the extreme route," wrote Buddy.[11]

For a night, anyway, Billy Carter was a Big Daddy of Plains unlike anything his father had ever embodied to the townsfolk. Friends and perfect strangers sat on whatever was available, including the floor, which was where Billy was to be found, livening up the tension from time to time by leading cheers laced with joyous profanity—"words not fittin' for the ears of a lady," as Beth Tartan recalled—as each state reported more and more votes favoring his brother. The hours went by, the food in the kitchen was grazed over and the alcohol imbibed again and again, and nerves were nearly shot as the news station reported that recounts were demanded or that counts were late or incomplete. It took Hawaii to save the day. At half past three in the morning, Plains time, CBS News reported that Jimmy had won the fiftieth state. "The Carter house rocked on its foundations," recalled Beth Tartan. Billy stripped off his shirt with a whoop and a holler. Underneath was a t-shirt bearing the slogan "Jimmy Won! '76"—obviously, Billy had been sure all along. But so had the rest of the Peanut Brigade. On the triple t.v. screens in Billy's living room, Lillian could be seen on the depot platform surrounded by members of the Brigade, all wearing the same shirt, samples of which were, in ambitious Carter fashion, available for sale (and at $4 apiece they soon sold out).[12]

Among the army of photographers in Plains that election day was a photojournalist named Steven Borns. A lean, bespectacled young man based in New York City but originally from Tampa, Borns had arrived in Plains in 1976 with the intention of doing a book solely about Lillian. Only after he got there did he realize that Plains itself amounted to more than just a marker on the map to show where Jimmy Carter was born.

Staying in the area a total of four months, and interviewing some seventy-five people, Borns' sojourn would result in *The People of Plains, GA*, his 1978 book of photographs and twenty-five interviews with many of the town's old timers. The book is a pictorial *Our Town* of the changing south, where comedy and majesty lived in every face and every life. Borns talked to everybody—to Rachel Clark, regal and forthright; to Hugh Carter, holding forth for hours about his worm farm; to his father Alton, who took Borns to the Carter family cemetery outside town and lectured him on Carter family history. School bus driver Staunton Shiver bared his soul in a soliloquy on a theme of integration, while Thomas and Eva Williams, the black proprietors of a dance club, declared they wanted to give it all up for Christ (and did). Borns also captured the fragile tracery of Ida Lee Timmerman, who had aided Earl Carter in secretly buying outfits for poor Plains children to wear to their high school graduation. Age and extreme delicacy of manner belied a soul as outraged by racism as Lillian's, showing that there was at least one other woman of her generation in town who was not comfortable with the status quo. Her perspective was so important to him and to the book, Borns says, he drove back to Plains to meet with her. And of course, Borns captured Lillian, too—or perhaps it would be more accurate to say that she captured him. She drove him around Plains, showing him the farmhouse at Archery and the fields of cotton and peanuts that flowed out in all directions. His single photograph of her in *The People of Plains* shows her sitting in a glow of maternal triumph, an elder Virgin Mary saucily informing the world, "I told you so"; on the screen is none other than Jimmy Carter, the success story of the decade, every mother's dream son.[13]

Lillian may have felt, as a mother has a right to do, that no success was a surprise where her son was concerned. But at the crowded election night depot, when the news of Jimmy Carter's win came through on Lillian's earpiece, the tension stiffening her every fiber disappeared. She stood, mouth open, just as surprised as everyone else was, and just as thrilled.

"None of it seemed real," wrote Beth Tartan. "A Danish newsman kept saying, 'Only in America could it happen.'"[14]

Billy had left his giant house-party and forced his way through glad-handing delirious crowds to where his mother stood on the platform. Holding a half-smoked cigarette, he jumped up beside her, laughing. With a brother who was President of the United States, the leader of the free world and head of the most powerful nation on earth, Billy was now officially The Other One, the clown prince of Plains, liquored up and loud and not for the last time. Lillian promptly, almost desperately, wrapped him in her arms.

"Just being on the fringes of fame does weird things to some people," wrote Buddy Carter. "You begin to think you're dusted with glitter or gold." Fame was to do weird things to Billy Carter, but it was also to do weird things to the entire Carter family. Lillian's reaching out to Billy on election night, the official start of four years of glitter and misery for the Carter family, begins to look less like a mother bringing her son close for a moment of supreme joy and more like a woman desperate to keep her child from flying away. Perhaps, too, she realized she needed someone to hold on to for the fast and very bumpy ride that was ahead for them both.[15]

CHAPTER 10

Believe

Jimmy Carter writes that among the superhuman challenges that faced him upon his inauguration was one no less pressing and very personal quandary—what to do with his mother.

It was obvious, he wrote, that Lillian "would be very active but had no staff or security." She would of course need protection for her visits to the White House (she had already staked out the Queen's Bedroom as her rightful territory). And the fact that she was still taking the bus to Atlanta once a month for meetings of the Department of Human Resources Board of Governors meant she would need protection in Georgia, too. But Lillian loved her independence. "Mama rejected any security for the first couple of months," wrote Jimmy Carter, "but then I decided that it would be necessary to include her as a member of my immediate family." This qualified her for the same level of twenty-four hour daily security that the First Family enjoyed, but would mean she would be tailed by Secret Service men in dark suits and ties. "This idea was abhorrent to Mama," recalled Carter. So he came up with a solution that pacified her and solved the problem. Georgia State Trooper Ray Hathcock, a burly man with a boyish face, was detailed by Georgia Governor George Busbee to serve as Lillian's bodyguard. "What started out as a security job turned into a personal aide job," Hathcock remembered.[1]

Where Lillian might have always felt uneasy in the presence of a stranger, Hathcock seemed like home folks. And he was the type of strong, good-looking man Lillian liked to have around, to joke and smoke and have a drink with. Hathcock eventually did her personal shopping for her, never letting her supply of Old Forester bourbon run low, and would even go to her favorite dress shops to pick up and pay for or return outfits chosen for her. He traveled the world by her side, occasionally serving as her prompter during speeches. Hathcock also came to know her temper very well. Lillian had a habit, increasing with age, of flying off the handle. This ranged from making statements to the press that everyone later wished they could reel back in, to sometimes abruptly firing long time household staff who knew to wait around until she rehired them an hour or so later.[2] Hathcock was present one day when Lillian unexpectedly ran into Hugh Carter, Jimmy's cousin. With a salesman's flair for timing, Carter had just published *Cousin Beedie and Cousin Hot*, his recollections of growing up with Jimmy and family in Plains, not a page of which missed a chance to share Carter family secrets or to get a dig into Lillian. And Lillian had read enough of it to know this. "She walked straight toward Hugh," remembered Hathcock, "and I got out of the way because I knew what was about to happen." According to Hugh, Lillian shouted at him, "You're the scum of the earth for what you said in your book about me." As Hathcock recalled, "Hugh just stood there grinning while taking it," grateful for publicity that would, of course, sell more copies of his book. Billy Carter later wrote that his mother and Hugh made peace before her death.[3]

With Hathcock in place, Jimmy Carter felt more assured about giving Lillian a more public presence, and within his first few months in the White House he was to test her in an international role.

As Jimmy Carter tells it, Lillian was sitting in the Pond House on February 11, 1977, and wondering what to do with herself when the phone rang. It was Jimmy, with news and a request. He first asked his mother how she was feeling. She needed to see her doctor, she said—she wasn't feeling too well. Jimmy asked, "How would you like to go to India?" Lillian replied that sure, someday she would love to go back. He then told her that Indian president Fakhruddin Ali Ahmed had died that day. And he asked, "'How about [going to India] this afternoon?'" She would be attending President Ali Ahmed's funeral as the Carter administration's representative—that is, if she felt up to it. By then, Lillian's ills, real or imagined, had evaporated. "I'll be ready," she told her son.[4]

Carter arranged for a plane to transport Lillian to Washington. She was met there by grandson Chip, who would be one of several people accompanying her overseas. "She said she didn't have anything to wear," recalled Jimmy, "and I promised that one of the stores in Washington would have a selection of black dresses waiting at the airport." This little black dress was to loom large over the next few hours.[5]

Rick Hutto was then working in the White House as appointments secretary to the First Family, and was brought in to coordinate logistics for Lillian's trip. Hutto and Lillian would develop the kind of affably close relationship she enjoyed with a number of men and an informality that on one occasion had Hutto fearing for his job. Hutto remembers the day well. Lillian was laid up in the Queen's Bedroom with a complaint that kept her bedridden and, having watched her soap operas, she was bored. She called Hutto to come keep her company—and to bring her a bottle of bourbon. Though the White House of the Carter administration was officially "dry," there was no refusing the First Mother. Hutto obliged by purchasing a bottle at a liquor store near the White House, which he then placed in its brown paper bag on Lillian's bedside table. They were sitting having a chat, recalls Hutto, when "I saw her look over my head, and she said, 'Hey, honey—come in!'" Hutto heard Jimmy Carter say, "How are you, Mama?," and when he turned saw the President "give a look at this brown bag on the nightstand. Then he looked at me. Then he looked back at her." Red-faced, Hutto excused himself and remembers sitting at his desk through the rest of the afternoon, sure that "within minutes I was going to be fired. But the President never said a word," he recalls.[6]

Now, on the eve of Lillian's departure for India, Hutto had another crisis to face down. She was already upset, Hutto says, because her favorite companion, Richard Harden, was unable to go with her. Harden was hard at work on the first year's budget, which had to be presented to Congress, and there was no way he could get away for a few days, even for her. Hutto points out that Lillian was not spoiled, she just knew with whom she felt most comfortable. She may have also guessed that the White House Press Secretary, Jody Powell, would want to assign her a minder on this first foray as presidential emissary. Lillian wasn't the only person upset; Powell was worried, too. "She had no hesitation about speaking her mind—sometimes early and often," remembers Rex Granum, deputy press secretary under Powell, "and there was some apprehension about what she might say on the trip."[7] Lillian and Powell had already had a bit of a tussle on her very first day at the White House. When Powell attempted to coach Lillian on how to respond to certain questions, she told him frankly to go to hell.[8] Harden would have made her feel more at ease and, most importantly, would also have been able to steer her clear of troubled waters.

"Miss Lillian was someone I had come to know well in the campaign," says Granum. "'There's nobody available to go from the First Lady's press office,' Jody Powell said to me. 'We sure can't send Miss Lillian by herself.' 'What about me?' I asked. 'You want to go to India?' he answered. 'I've *been* to Plains,' I said. 'I haven't *been* to India. Sure.'" Granum, in fact, was

Lillian's "second favorite," and the decision to send him with her helped ameliorate her disappointment that he wasn't Richard Harden. "We got along extremely well," Granum recalls. Once Lillian's situation was sorted out, the rest of the plans fell into place: Sen. Charles Percy of Illinois and his wife and freshman Congressman John Kavanagh from Nebraska, as well as a State Department specialist, Adolph "Spike" Dubs, were included among the delegation. Everything was set except for what would seem the insignificant detail of what to wear to the funeral.[9]

Hutto remembers when the call came from "some officious clerk in the State Department." The woman gave him a list of to-dos to give to Lillian. "And she explicitly told me to tell Miss Lillian that she needed to bring a black dress to wear to the Indian president's funeral," says Hutto. He relayed the list to an increasingly impatient First Mother, "who chafed at being told what to do—though she really did want to do the right thing, of course," says Hutto. "But when I got to the part about needing to bring a black dress, she hit the roof. She said, 'And embarrass our country and embarrass my son?' I asked what she meant. She said, '*White* is the color of mourning in India. If I were to step off the plane in a black dress I would be insulting the entire country.'" White, she explained, was the color worn by Indian widows, the color worn to mark a death in the family. To Lillian, the Indian people were family. She would wear white to join them in mourning the death of their president and show India that Americans respected their customs, something she knew better about than some "officious" State Department clerk.[10] However, though she did step off the plane wearing white, international protocol seems to have stepped in to settle the matter of what she wore to the funeral itself. Mrs. Gandhi would be wearing a white sari; perhaps because it was deemed improper for the mother of the United States president to wear the same color as the Indian prime minister, Lillian ended up wearing a black dress, and this clearly rankled in her well after the trip was over. As Jimmy Carter recalls, a few weeks after his mother returned home she called him, furious, to say that she had received a bill for the dress, which she had not even wanted to wear in the first place.[11]

Rex Granum remembers the flight well. "Miss Lillian, of course, took the forward area where a president would normally be," he says. "She did treat the funeral quite seriously and was determined to represent her country quite properly. But there was no getting around the fact that she was ecstatic to be going back to a country she loved so much. And presumably in slightly better style than when she first went!"[12] When Air Force Two landed in Teheran for refueling, Lillian got off to greet the base commander, who rolled out the red carpet for his visitors. "Large portions of caviar were brought on the plane." Granum recalls. "This was some two years before the hostage crisis, which tells you how quickly things change." Lillian's good mood only got better when, as the plane rose into the air again, a call was put through to Lillian from President Carter. "At Rosalynn's suggestion, I told [her] that I could have the plane stop at Bombay after the funeral," Carter wrote, "if Mother wanted to visit the site of her Peace Corps work." Not only was Rosalynn's suggestion a brilliant one in terms of Indo-American relations, it was also an extremely thoughtful gesture toward Lillian.[13]

Lillian was still on a cloud when she stepped off the plane in New Delhi. "The Indian government had set up a very large tent adjacent to the runway," says Granum, "so that the arriving delegations from various countries could be greeted at the airport." As head of the American delegation, Lillian was met in the tent by Prime Minister Indira Gandhi. This was a

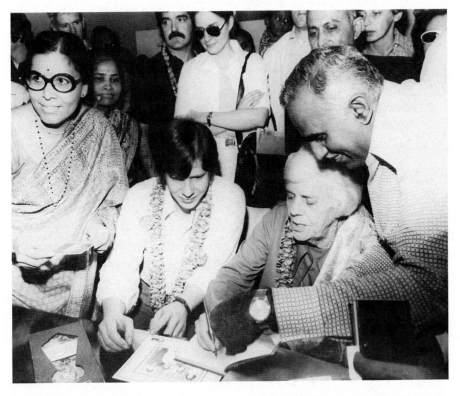

Lillian, seated with grandson Chip Carter, signs a copy of her book *Away From Home: Letters to My Family* **as friends look on (courtesy Peace Corps)**

delicate encounter to be sure, since Lillian had never been a fan of Mrs. Gandhi's during or after her time in India. The previous October, Lillian had publicly criticized Gandhi's government for what she believed was diversion of food aid by government officials away from the poor who most needed it. She later claimed she was misquoted, but she had so freely shared this opinion of Gandhi's government that few believed her. Whatever was said in the welcome tent, according to Rex Granum, it obviously worked wonders. "Here is Miss Lillian with her arm around Indira Gandhi, and vice versa, coming out of the tent and walking to our much smaller group of staff," Granum remembers. "Miss Lillian comes over to me and in that deep, wonderful South Georgia accent, says, '*Wrecks*, I'd like yah tah meet In-deer-uh. In-deer-uh, *Wrecks*'!' [Granum's phonetics] I mumbled something like, 'Very nice to meet you, Madame Prime Minister.'"[14] Later on, Gandhi and Lillian reappeared from a more private meeting in the prime minister's residence after what was described in the press as a forty-five minute "very lovely social meeting." Lillian was careful to tell reporters that "I came out of there admiring her very much and my whole opinion of her changed."[15]

At President Ali Ahmed's funeral, Lillian laid a wreath at the bier, alongside that brought by Prince Michael of Kent, emissary of Queen Elizabeth II, and performed her duties with dignity. She then headed for Bombay and Vikhroli, where Rex Granum had preceded her with a USIS press attaché. "He and I flew down ahead," Granum remembers, "to make sure everything was arranged. Not that we had to set anything up or choreograph anything, because the people in Bombay had everything well in hand." Granum still remembers how thrilled Lillian was. "She was just over the moon to be back among the people for whom she had cared," he says. "I think it's possible she thought she would never get to see them again. So it was very emotional for her."[16]

"I can't wait to kiss everybody," Lillian told a reporter.[17]

With Chip Carter and an entourage of Americans at her side, Lillian arrived in the Godrej complex wearing an elegant green outfit. But her friends were nowhere to be seen. "She was embarrassed and crestfallen when no one was there to meet her," wrote Jimmy Carter. Making the best of the situation, Lillian guided her brood along a street where she had walked many times in bare feet, telling them she wanted to show them the location of her old apartment at 13/6 Godrej Hillside Colony. "When they made the turn," Carter wrote, "there were more than ten thousand people waiting in complete silence," who burst into applause and cheers as Lillian appeared.[18]

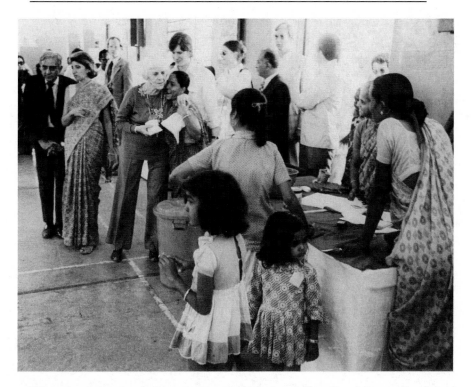

When she returned to India in 1977 as First Mother, Lillian found thousands of people waiting to greet her (courtesy Peace Corps).

Carmen Kagal of SPAN Magazine watched America's First Mother, her neck draped in flowers, as she sat listening to welcome speeches. "Like a searchlight her gaze sweeps across the crowd, looking for familiar faces," wrote Kagal. "As she spots them, she smiles, she waves, she blows kisses." Between the towering green spires of *ashoka* trees, the "sorrow-less" tree associated with the Hindu god of love and traditionally the tree under which the Buddha was born, "stretches a dense mass of heads, mostly male workers. A scattering of women. Children in festive garb." When it came time for Lillian to approach the dais to address the crowd, she appeared overcome by the applause. She put her hands over her streaming face, dabbed at her eyes with Kleenex, and managed to recover enough to speak. "Everywhere I have been since I left here, I have spoken of my love for Vikhroli—not just India, but Vikhroli," she told the crowd. "I love every one of you. Thank you for coming."[19]

The emotional journey continued. Lillian visited the dispensary and had a reunion with Dr. Bhatia and the male nurse Raja, who had seen her

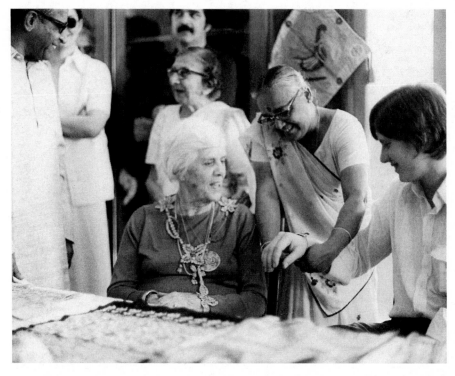

Lillian looks on as a sacred thread is tied around Chip Carter's wrist, celebrating the visit (courtesy Peace Corps)

off at the airport in 1968. They lovingly placed a silk shawl around her shoulders. Dr. Bhatia was still working long hours at the clinic, and he filled her in on all the latest news. She was delighted to greet one of her favorite patients, an Untouchable man named Shri Nath, who a decade before had suffered badly from asthma. Lillian took him in her arms, and when she heard that Shri Nath's condition had improved markedly, she announced to everyone in the room, "But of course. *I* cured him!"[20]

Lillian was not an easy weeper in public—she had been dry-eyed at her son's swearing in as president, surely an occasion when a woman was allowed to bawl in front of God and everybody. But she wept many happy tears on this visit, especially when she saw what improvements had been made at the clinic. The hospital she had been consulted for in 1967 was in process of being built by the Godrej family, and Lillian felt that in some way she had played a role in making it a reality. Yet she shrank from praise for her work. As when she was in Vikhroli, all she wanted was to be useful and to help people who had no one else to help them. Visiting patients in a hospital with nurses guiding her, Lillian was overheard to say, "I feel like an angel, but I know I'm not." Jimmy Carter writes that on his mother's return he shared with her a State Department report on her trip. Lillian's return to India "was a superb diplomatic effort," Carter was informed, "and that we had the best relations now with India that we'd had since 1960, largely because of her visit and her obvious concern for the Indian people." If that wasn't being an angel, it was surely next door to one.[21]

It wasn't just her friends in India that Lillian wanted to reach out and embrace. She tried to keep in touch with her fellow Peace Corps volunteers. She sought out Mabel Yewell, who by 1977 was living in a convalescent home in Bel Air, Maryland. Mabel had never really recovered from the experience of working in Vikhroli for two years. In fact, she had returned from India in even worse shape than Lillian, if that was possible. While in Vikhroli, Mabel had contracted amoebic dysentery, bronchitis, asthma "and everything else," she told a reporter later. In her final years she was bedridden and living in Bel Air Convalescent Center. Lillian was driven seventy miles from Washington to spend an hour with her, bringing "greetings and flowers from the White House," according to a press report. She arrived wearing a stylish blue suit and seeming many years Mabel's junior. She was also in a teasing mood. "All the good things you've heard about me are true," she quipped as she greeted the Center's patients, "all the bad things are lies." She and Mabel "yacked," according to Mabel, as they had done years before in 13/6 Godrej Hillside Colony, but the visit was brief because Lillian had to rush back to the White House for a meeting. When asked if she and Lillian planned to see each other again, it was frail Mabel's turn to deliver a wisecrack. "If we're both on deck," she said, "I'll see her soon, if not then I won't." Mabel died a little over a year later, on May 10, 1978, and Lillian wrote to her family that her passing "grieves me a lot."[22]

Larry Brown, who went on to work with the Peace Corps in Washington, D.C., was another volunteer Lillian tracked down. During the presidential campaign, Brown visited her at the Pond House. "I got a rental car in Atlanta and drove to Plains," recalls Brown. "I had to ask twice where Miss Lillian lived, and both times the people I happened to stop knew exactly. The town did have several people around who looked interested in all the goings on, who I took to be Secret Service." Two other "locals" showed Brown where the house was, and there Lillian met him at the door. Brown had brought her lobsters from Boston, where he was then living, which they prepared in her kitchen. "The next night, Lilly returned the favor by cooking me a Georgia ham, about the saltiest meat I ever ate," Brown recalls. "I told her it made me pucker so much I couldn't talk, and she laughed and said maybe it ought to be served in Congress."[23]

Lillian made Brown a part of her life in Plains by taking him with her to greet tourists at the train depot and also to church services of a Sunday. "I remember no details of what she was saying to me during the service," he recalls, "only that what she said was funny or gossipy. It probably bored Lilly as much as it did me, so she was like a kid in Sunday school." Along with this, Lillian shared with Brown some of what her life as First Mother and popular icon was like. After the Carters had moved into the White House, she would call Brown at the Peace Corps offices to invite him over. "I'd walk up to the front of the White House gate, they'd look at my ID, and send me through unescorted to the living quarters," he remembers. "Sometimes Lilly would be right there, and sometimes I'd look around the unoccupied rooms until she arrived. Once she showed me the Lincoln Bedroom, pushing me down on the bed until I was prone, saying, 'Now isn't that a nice bed, Abe?' And on another visit she had me sit on the floor with her, Indian style, to talk." While they sat there, sipping red wine, Andrew J. Young arrived "and joined us for several minutes of chit-chat." Brown enjoyed taking part in her charmed life.[24]

Back when Jimmy was Governor of Georgia, Lillian had sent repeated invitations to Gabe and Ruth Ross, the Peace Corps volunteers to whom she had sent *The Prophet* in India, to come see her. They were then living in Philadelphia. "Our house was on a hill," remembers Ruth, "and the only time the mailman came up the driveway was to deliver a Christmas card from Plains, Georgia—later it said 'The White House.' He would hand carry these things up to our apartment." In her cards and notes, Lillian complained that the Rosses never came to visit her. "She invited us to come to the Governor's Mansion," says Gabe. "It's foolish, but we never accepted. We were poor, I was in grad school, and maybe there were reasons related to the whole Southern thing." They were of the opinion of many liberal thinkers north of the Mason-Dixon Line: that the south was a place of tyranny for all but white good old boys, and not a safe place for people of very different beliefs, social and religious.[25]

Still, the Rosses had followed Jimmy Carter's career enough to know that he was not cut from that cloth. On the night he was nominated at the Democratic Convention in New York City, Ruth decided she would call the Americana Hotel, where she knew the Carters were staying, to give her and Gabe's congratulations. "I asked to speak to Lilly, and somebody put her on the phone," Ruth remembers. "I said, 'Lilly, I can't believe that Jimmy is really going to be nominated tonight!' And Lilly went into a complete non sequitur like, 'Do you know that Carol [Stahl, a Peace Corps volunteer] dyed her hair blond?'" Ruth couldn't get her to veer away from gossip about the other Peace Corps volunteers, "and who had visited her and whom she'd visited ... absolutely downplaying the fact that her son was going to be nominated that night."[26]

In Jimmy's first year as president, the Rosses received an invitation that they did accept, to a Peace Corps reunion in Washington. The setting was a hotel not far from the White House, followed by a state dinner at the mansion. "We were excited about this opportunity," says Gabe, "even though the President was not going to be there—he was at an economic conference in Bonn." After they settled into their hotel, and met up with a few volunteers they had not seen since the 1960s, the Rosses joined the other invitees on a stroll to the White House. "We entered the State Dining Room," says Gabe, "and there was Lilly with the Indian ambassador. There were all kinds of neat, interesting people around. And we had a wonderful time—the dinner, the tour through the grounds, just incredible. I think it was all the more so for us because Ruth and I are foreign-born," explains Gabe. "Ruth was born in Germany and I was born in Kazakhstan, which was then part of the Soviet Union. Our parents are Holocaust survivors and we were brought here as immigrants. Yet here we were at the White House!"[27]

The Rosses didn't have much of an opportunity to speak with Lillian at the dinner, except for one brief but significant exchange. "We were all dressed up, and I was wearing a silver necklace," Ruth says. "Lilly came up to me and showed me her necklace. It was the Hebrew word, *chai*, which is the symbol for the number eighteen, a spiritual number in Judaism. A good luck symbol. My necklace had the same symbol on it. Lilly said, in her drawl, 'Ruth, mah *chai* is nicer than *your chai*.' I said, 'Where did you get your *chai*?' She replied, 'Menachem Begin gave it to me.' I didn't think she knew what a *chai* was!"[28]

Gabe and Ruth thought that might be it, and it was certainly more than they expected. But at the Peace Corps conference the next day, in the middle of one of the sessions, "all of a sudden, Lilly comes over to me," recalls Gabe, "and says, 'Gabe, you're a strange individual!'" She reiterated what she had written in her many notes delivered up the hill in Philadelphia: how she had asked him and Ruth to come to Plains, and to Atlanta, and now to Washington, "but you didn't even respond, outside of Christmas wishes!" Now that she had them captive, as it were, Lillian insisted on showing the Rosses a good time. "Would you and Ruth be interested in coming to the White House with me?" She asked Gabe to find out if Ruth, who was at another session, might be interested in the visit. "I can't sneak a group of people in with me," Lillian explained, "so don't tell anybody else." Gabe said, "Of course, we'd love to. I'll go find Ruth. Where shall we meet you?" Before disappearing back into the crowd, Lillian said, "Just in front of the hotel there'll be a limo waiting. And we'll go have lunch at the White House."[29]

Gabe and Ruth emerged from the hotel not entirely sure what to expect. But there was the limousine, and in it was Lillian, with Secret Service men standing nearby. As the car glided through the gates of the Executive Mansion and took them to a private entrance near the back of the complex, the Rosses thought with amusement of all the ID checking they had gone through the evening before, totally dispensed with now. "We were soon upstairs," Gabe recalls. Lillian gave them a tour of the area. "This is the Lincoln Bedroom," she told them, "this is Jimmy and Rosalynn's bedroom, and there's Amy's. There's my bedroom when I'm here. And there's where President Nixon dropped an ash from his cigar the night before he resigned from the presidency—see the mark on the carpet? It's still there." Gabe and Ruth remember entering the private dining room where Chip Carter, his wife and infant son were sitting having lunch and to whom they were introduced. "Lilly then introduced us to the chef," Ruth remembers, "and asked us what we wanted to eat. A wonderful lunch was served."[30]

After the meal, Lillian told the Rosses that she had a few pressing things she had to do, and wouldn't be away for long. In the meantime, did they want to stay a bit and have a look around? "Well!" exclaims Gabe. "All of a sudden, we're alone in the White House! So we went back over all these rooms, doing what anybody else in our position might want to do— we lay on the President's bed, we opened the little nightstand to see what he was reading; we used the bathroom." Ruth ventured out to the Truman balcony, where she waved to tourists lined up below. "People started waving back," she says. "They must have thought I was Rosalynn or somebody!"[31]

Because an hour had passed and Lillian was still nowhere to be seen, the Rosses ended up in her bedroom, sitting on her bed, asking each other if all this could really be happening, when they heard what they thought was Lillian in a room down the hall. They investigated, found the door of the President's private study ajar, and pushed it open. They saw not Lillian but "some guy working on his knees, who stands up and says, 'Gabby!' and grabs me." It was Joseph Klechevsky, nicknamed Jossi, whom Gabe had known since Jossi was fourteen, having met him at a secular Jewish camp of which Gabe was director. Born in Poland after the Holocaust, Jossi had gone to Israel, then come to the United States, and was working for a high fidelity company. As the Rosses soon discovered, this was why Jossi was at the White House, setting up a hi-fi system for the President, who had a deep love of classical music. "When he came to the U.S., he couldn't speak English," Gabe explains, "and here he was at the White House!" They gathered at the grand piano in the Center Hall and with Gabe at the keyboard began to belt out old camp songs in Yiddish. Then they realized they were being watched. The technicians whom Jossi supervised were standing there in amazement that their boss knew somebody who was in the White House, "and was singing with him in Yiddish, yet!" After another hour or so, Lillian returned and asked, "Did you all have a good time?" Yes, Gabe and Ruth told her, exchanging smiles, they had indeed.[32]

In March 1978, Lillian made clear that she was prepared to get involved in the ongoing problem of world hunger. In a speech given that month at a UNICEF fundraiser in Chicago, at which she received an award, she said, "I learned while serving with the Peace Corps in India that one of the most basic human rights is the right to have food.... After a year of watching, I have decided to give my son some help in dealing with this problem of world hunger. What am I going to do? I intend to work with people like you who are already actively involved. I intend to speak out on the problem and encourage others to do likewise. I intend to meet with political and business leaders to ask them what they are doing to try to help solve the problem. I intend to help focus attention on the projects that have been successful.... It is my hope that the historians will say that my son set us on the course that eventually led to a 'world without hunger.'"[33]

Lillian's biggest effort to address world hunger actually began very quietly with the news that she had been awarded the Ceres medal by the Director-General of the Food and Agriculture Organization of the United Nations. Since 1971, the FAO had bestowed the Ceres medal annually to celebrate the work of women in social justice and agricultural development. Lillian was to be given the medal for her work for civil rights in her community and for her Peace Corps service in India. She seemed embarrassed or at least puzzled by the award at first, but said that if Jimmy and his National Security Advisor Zbigniew Kazimierz Brzezinski approved, she would accept it. They did approve. Her craggy portrait, sculpted by Frank Gasparro, was featured on one side of the medal while the other bore words which Lillian chose—"Human kindness and caring heal beyond any wall"—

and the faces of three nurses displaying characteristics of three different ethnicities.[34]

According to Richard Harden, Dr. Peter Bourne, who served President Carter as special assistant for health issues, had merely asked that Lillian come up from Plains to receive the medal in Washington in a special ceremony. Harden suggested that they go one better and arrange for her to receive the award in Rome, where it was traditionally given at the FAO offices facing the Palatine Hill. "We then decided that if she was in Rome, she could have a trip to visit less fortunate people in West Africa," Harden says. As it happened, the President of Gambia, Al Hadji Sir Dawda Jawara, came to Plains in person to invite Lillian to visit the Sahel region. On a rainy late spring day, the Gambian president and a retinue of thirteen drove out to the Pond House, where Lillian greeted them with a happiness in part due to the welcome last minute parting of rain clouds. As they both sat on the living room sofa, the president in his colorful robes and Lillian in one of her now-famous pale pantsuits, Sir Dawda Jawara handed her his invitation to visit his nation. Not only did Lillian show the Gambian delegation around her country retreat, but they were able to go to Plains and meet people there. "That visit to your country was also very rewarding," the president said in a speech on Lillian's arrival in Africa later that summer, "in that it permitted me and my delegation to meet and discuss with a significant portion of the Black Community in America and to further strengthen the already very solid contacts that exist between us."[35]

What the Gambian president wanted Lillian to see was the drought conditions in the Sahel Region, which had been an ongoing concern since the late 1960s. Based on this invitation, says Richard Harden, "the State Department then built an itinerary that would include Senegal, Mali and Upper Volta." In tandem with this, it was arranged for Lillian to meet representatives from the Club du Sahel in Paris, the association founded in 1976 to bring together Sahelian states affected by the drought, at the Organization for Economic Cooperation and Development in Paris. So this made France the first stop of her tour. Far from being merely a progress to Rome to receive the Ceres medal, Lillian was now making a trip of far broader scope and intention, as an emissary for her son and to "express the president's deep interest in the problem of world hunger, the disparity between the rich and poor, and the role of women in the development process."[36]

She had a grueling schedule of ahead of her: Gambia from July 24 to 26, Senegal from July 26 to 28, Upper Volta from July 28 to 31, and Mali from July 31 to August 2. She would return home a week and five days before her eightieth birthday, which raised the question of whether she was taking on too much for a woman her age. Lillian laughed off the concern, telling reporters "I anticipate living a long time. I'm going to complete what I started before I go."[37]

That Lillian had a deep interest in the region herself is evident in comments she made to the press. As she told a reporter from *The Afro-American*, "I have heard about all these things about the Sahel, but I haven't seen them.... Don't get mad, but I have to see to believe."[38] One member of her entourage, Arthur Fell, had already seen the route she would be taking in Africa. "We first went to check everything out," he said in a 1997 interview, "then I had to go back a second time when we actually made the trip with her." Fell found her an interesting person, curious about those who were accompanying her. She told him during the trip, "I'd like to know more of what you're thinking." Fell shared with her his hopes for USAID, the African Bureau of which Fell had joined in 1969, moving the organization's mission to Senegal in 1975. Right at the time of Lillian's trip, Fell said, "we were trying to 'sell' the Sahel program and to encourage the administration to do as much as we could for those countries and to keep the network we were trying to build going." His main fear was that "the United States would just lose heart and pull out." They didn't, he pointed out. Likely his responses to Lillian's questions about what he wanted to do in Africa were taken, like the appeals from Georgians in need, directly to her son's desk, with an urgent suggestion that he do something about it.[39]

In Paris, Lillian was briefed for two hours by members of the Club du Sahel on the challenges faced by the region. As usual, she pushed through the abstracts of regional issues to the individuals on whom drought and famine had a direct impact. "I will meet the people in the villages," she told the press. "The common people—that's who I want to meet. That's what I've been doing all my life. I don't strive to meet heads of state," though she had to bend that rule by having tea with Mme Valéry Giscard d'Estaing, wife of the French president.[40]

Lillian moved on to Rome, where she received her Ceres medal from FAO Director Eduard Saoma "with a broad smile." In her remarks, she again paid tribute to ordinary people by drawing attention to the larger forces that affected their lives and could, if used properly, improve their lives. Her speech given at the event offered as prime example her own place on the continuum:

> I come from a part of the United States in which agriculture is vitally important and now highly mechanized. It was not always this way as you know. I was fortunate to live at a time when electric power reached our community,

when the fruits of important scientific research were made available to us, when my children were able to receive full public school educations. These things: electricity, education, applied scientific research in agriculture and a lot of hard work changed our lives in a kind of peaceful revolution. We were able to make our lives more comfortable, our community more prosperous, and to look beyond it to others less fortunate. If these fundamental changes in the life of our family had not occurred in those days I would not have had the opportunity or the inspiration or even the time to join the Peace Corps and serve in a village in India—where people just as we did are striving to better their lives by learning to apply new methods of health, of family planning, of farming.

"The world cannot afford the waste that derives from too much pride," she concluded, "from competition or distrust between nations…. Through all of you and with you we must create that same peaceful revolution of the farms and in the villages of the world that made it possible for me to receive today this honor in this beautiful, eternal, city of Rome."[41]

Again, heads of state had to be met, and as she so often did, Lillian's informality and directness charmed the presidents and kings she insisted on treating like everybody else. She paid a visit to the recently elected Socialist Alessandro Pertini, President of Italy, who at eighty-one was two years her senior. To the delight of the press corps and of Pertini, Lillian referred to the elderly leader as "your new young president."[42] After Lillian's arrival, Pertini asked her if she had any advice to share with him for the next seven years of his term. "Just do what you have been doing all your life," she said, "fighting for human rights and helping the poor." This so charmed Pertini that he replied to Lillian, when she asked what he would like her to take back to her son, that President Carter "should follow the example of his mother in her concern to alleviate hunger and hardship." When they bade each other goodbye, they had found much in common. "You are like me," Pertini told Lillian. "You say what is on your mind and in your heart." U.S. Ambassador Richard N. Gardner declared himself thrilled with Lillian's diplomacy in her meeting with President Pertini. "Miss Lillian made a profound impression on President Pertini," recalled Gardner. "'Listening to Mrs. Carter,' he said, 'I felt I was hearing my own mother.'"[43]

Lillian also had an audience with Pope Paul VI at his summer residence on Lake Como—one of the last he ever gave, since the pontiff died only two weeks later. During the meeting, which lasted for twenty-five minutes, First Mother met Holy Father and quipped later to reporters, "Being in the presence of a man so holy made me feel holy too." But Lillian took the meeting very seriously, declaring that it was "the most moving moment in my life." The Pope was a little over a year older than Lillian but in poor health, yet this fragility seemed only to underscore what she saw as his remarkable gentleness.[44] The Pope had just given a speech to a crowd of thousands assembled below the balcony of Castel Gandolfo in which he appealed for aid for famine- and war-stricken Ethiopia and Eritrea.[45] In a letter, Lillian described how the Pope greeted her in his office and graciously accepted President Carter's letter. He listened as she told him she was on her way to some of the most drought-ravaged areas of Africa and asked if he would pray for rain. Before Lillian departed, the Pope confided to Lillian that as he was old and tired, he was fully prepared to "go to the arms of God." Lillian replied, "Holy Father, if you go before I do, will you tell him about me?" His Holiness promised to do so if Lillian promised to do the same should she go before he did. She was not slow to point out that as soon as she reached the Sahel, it rained and did not stop all the time she was there. "I am not Catholic," Lillian wrote, "but I am sure that this was no coincidence.[46]

From Rome to Africa meant a rest stop along the way. Lillian's plane landed in Rabat, Morocco, where she sipped mint tea with Princess Lalla Aicha, sister of King Hassan II, in a cool room that looked as if it had been created out of sheets of delicate wooden lace. She met the king himself, too, which later led to a characteristically comic exchange. King Hassan's offer of a case of rare perfumes was declined, says Jimmy Carter, because Lillian told the king she didn't have room in her luggage. After her return home in August, she arrived in Washington in time for the king's state visit. The king was given the Lincoln Bedroom, which put him across the hall from Lillian in the Queen's Bedroom. At the formal state dinner that night the two chatted like old friends; after dinner, the king invited her to his room, where he placed in her hands a vial of perfume, offering her the entire case again. She declined as she had done in Rabat, saying, "You damn foreigners are all alike!" But she took a royal kiss on the cheek.[47]

Pulitzer Prize-winning photographer Moneta Sleet, Jr., was sent by *Ebony* and *Jet* magazines (the latter was, by Lillian's admission, "my favorite ... I read it all the time") to document the African leg of Lillian's trip. (Afterward, it would be pointed out to the American press by Tom Smith, West African Affairs director for the State Department, that aside from this coverage, they had "all but ignored the trip.")[48] Sleet joined Lillian's entourage in Rome, which now included Rep. Cardiss Collins of Illinois and Rep. Charles W. Whalen of Ohio, and remained throughout the Morocco stop and the visits to the Sahel. *Ebony*'s editors wrote that while they would have preferred sending both a photographer and journalist, Sleet's reportage was as keenly observant as his camera. Indeed, through his lens, the world would watch as Lillian met the leaders of each nation, including the portly Nada Moro, Emperor of Mossi in Ouagadougou, Upper Volta (now Burkina Faso), descended staircases on the arms of presidents and stood to attention for gun salutes, posed in evening gowns in rooms filled with gilded furniture and velvet upholstery, sampled African delicacies with state officials in Mali. In Dakar she met Dr. Marie-Thérèse Basse, the first female doctor in Senegal, and they bantered like old friends, and she posed with the strikingly beautiful Mme Lena Gueye, vice president of the Senegalese National Assembly, holding her hand with what was for Lillian the rare expression of wordless joy. She visited artists, one of whom, Kaodima Lamourdia, director of the National Art Center of Upper Volta, presented her with her portrait. She met a little Malian girl, Sira Sissoko, who gave her a bouquet of flowers in the presence of U.S. Ambassador to Mali Patricia Byrne. (Like Madhavi Pethe, the Indian girl in whom Lillian took an interest in Vikhroli who grew up to be a university president, Sissoko grew up to have a professional career as an artist.) After meeting Caroline Diop, Senegal's minister of social action, Lillian wrote her a warm note that included these words: "It was a special pleasure for me to be accompanied by such a dynamic, concerned and politically alive woman as yourself." And Lillian made time to speak to Peace Corps volunteers in every place she visited; one image from the trip shows her seated on a chair in a village common area while young people sit at her feet, drinking in the humor and wisdom she is so clearly imparting. As a former Volunteer, she knew that though the nation of which her son was executive sent millions of dollars each year to fund relief programs in areas like the Sahel, none of it mattered if there weren't capable boots on the ground and people to stand in them whose passion was to help those in need without any desire for recompense. "I know that whatever happens in those countries," Lillian commented later, "the presence and work of the volunteers is critical in making it happen."[49]

The most important aspect of the trip that people saw through Sleet's eyes were the people themselves—the real reason Lillian had come to the villages, to meet the individuals who filled the streets and fields. "Miss Lillian Carter's trip through the drought-ravaged Sahel region of Africa was a stunning success," wrote Sleet, "because the 80-year old mother of President Carter was very willing and able to touch the people there, both rich and poor."[50]

Lillian's first stop after Rabat was Gambia, where roads were lined with crowds shouting "Welcome Miss Lillian." After meeting with President Sir Dawda Jawara in the capital, Banjul, where the president remarked, "You bring us two gifts we won't forget—your visit and rain"— Lillian boarded the presidential yacht and headed up the Gambia River for the town of Juffure, her delegation following in smaller boats.[51]

In 1976, author Alex Haley made history and helped start a craze for genealogical research with the publication of *Roots: The Saga of an American Family*. His novelized account of an eighteenth century ancestor from Gambia named Kunta Kinte captivated millions of readers. Kidnapped and delivered to the trans–Atlantic slave trade, Kunta Kinte became Toby Reynolds and lived out his life on a southern plantation but never forgot the culture or the spirit of Africa. In Juffure, the home of the Kinte clan, Haley was treated like a cross between a long lost son and a returning warrior, and the fame of his book and the television miniseries and sequels that spun off from it brought the boons and burdens of fame to the village much as Jimmy Carter's presidency was to do to Plains.

As she was guided up Gambian dirt roads in summer 1978, Lillian must have sympathized with the people of Juffure for reasons other than why she was there. They were used by now to *Roots*-related tourism and world attention, but not a delegation of this size or international prestige. With Lillian, who was steadied over the rough ground by the arm of President Al Hadji Sir Dawda Jawara of Gambia, came a retinue of journalists, American politicians, White House staff (including her favorite traveling companion, Richard Harden), tramping into the village like an invading army. Surely somewhere in Juffure, where as in Plains the cash registers were ringing a happy tune, was an elderly woman not unlike herself, longing for all the madness to stop.

"The heavy rains, which gave temporary relief from the drought, had muddied the roads," reported Sleet; a doctor in the entourage worried about Lillian's ability to cope with the jouncing journey to the town. "But Miss Lillian was undeterred," wrote Sleet. He was at Lillian's side when she entered Juffure, where she was greeted "by hundreds of people, among them being 78-year-old Benta Kinte, the matriarch of the Kinte family," who gave her her white robe as a gift of high respect. While she was in the village, Lillian spoke to the villagers, as she had promised to do in Rome, standing in a palm-roofed open pavilion while dozens of Juffurians, and the ubiquitous press corps, gathered around to listen. She planted a tree in honor of the visit, then visited what Sleet called a "slave house." This may have been the remains of a slave station called James Island, dating from the colonial period, located not far from Juffure, which itself owed its existence to a combination of native African and foreign (Portuguese and English) influence. The whole area had played a role in the trans–Atlantic slave trade, with Africans helping Europeans enslave members of rival tribal groups—such was the history behind Alex Haley's family and *Roots*, and indeed, the history of the Carters and Gordys, who had benefited from slavery before the Civil War.[52]

Past injustices were, however, not the focus of the journey, but the more immediate injustices Third World poor experienced daily throughout their often short lives. As she had done in India, from the day she set foot in Africa Lillian involved herself directly with ordinary people. She talked to mothers, caressing their babies and asking about their diet, their medical care, what they needed most and what they hoped for from the future. In one village she was photographed trying out a *pilon*, the heavy wooden pestle nearly as tall as she was with which African women pounded millet, giving up after the first few strokes. And she visited hospitals, including a leprosarium in Mali. "I saw children with their hands clenched and men with their hands clenched," she told Sleet, and was amazed by the local doctor's ability to reverse some of the symptoms. "To have a young boy with clenched hands straighten out every finger," she marveled. "That touched me.... And that's the only time I went home at night and cried." She also wept, she said, for all the children who were not so lucky as these. Seeing whole families of people living with leprosy, who had this hope of at least some recovery, who were "dancing and happy," was for Lillian "the most outstanding thing" on her trip.[53]

Twenty years later, Lillian's great-grandson, Georgia state senator and gubernatorial candidate Jason Carter, went to South Africa in 1998 with the Peace Corps, eager to follow in her footsteps. He met there a woman of strength and inspiration called Gogo—Zulu for "grandmother"—who like the matriarch who was his great-grandmother taught him more about life through the endurance with which she met each day's struggles than anyone else during his two years of service. "In Gogo's mind," Carter wrote in his memoir, *Power Lines*, "she translated the word 'hope' to the Zulu word *themba*. '*Themba*' means not only 'hope' but also 'believe.' For Gogo, 'hope' is not a possibility but a certainty. Too often, perhaps, we lose hope because we fail to look for it where we least expect it—among poor black people in a South African homeland or an American inner city, or poor white farmers in clapboard shacks in south Georgia. But there it is."[54]

His other Gogo, Miss Lillian, had already helped show him the way.

CHAPTER 11

Mixed Blessings

To say that Lillian lived a life she could not have possibly imagined or prepared for is an understatement.

Looking back over the last few years of Lillian Carter's life, Rex Granum is still impressed by the verve with which an elderly woman from rural south Georgia, well traveled though she was, handled the harsh spotlight trained on her every move after her son was elected president. "That was not something you could reasonably put in your life game plan," he says. "All of that occurred late in her life, and to her great joy, in my opinion."[1]

Like celebrities of stage, screen, sports or politics, Lillian became a regular on talk shows, especially The Tonight Show with Johnny Carson. On June 21, 1979, Carson asked her, "Do you know whether the President ever watches this show?" Lillian, seated beside Carson's desk wearing a sea-green silk dress and sparkling with delight, said, "Yes, he does. He's going to watch this one!" Hiding her face dramatically, she then looked directly into the camera and said, "Jimmy, I'm sorry!" When Carson wanted to know whether Carter ever asked for her advice, Lillian insisted he did not and that she never offered. "I think he knows more about the world than I do," she said. "I'll tell you another thing," she added. "Jimmy knows I speak whatever I want to. He never criticizes me. He likes everything I do." The studio roared with applause, as they did when she appeared on the Dinah Shore Show in November 1978. Telling Shore about her trip to Africa, Lillian regaled her and the audience with descriptions of visiting Timbuktu with an escort of six hundred elephants. "Ray [Hathcock] rode an elephant," she drawled, "and I smelled him for a week afterward." At the funeral of Pope John Paul I, she told Shore, she was asked which of the attendant cardinals she would choose as his successor. The Vatican official probably didn't expect her response any more than Shore's audience did. She told him she liked the "good looking one" standing off to one side, who turned out to be Pope John Paul II (canonized on Sunday, April 27, 2014). "And they chose him!" she said with an awe that did not fool her audience but certainly delighted them. Perhaps her crowning prime time moment was when, as guest of Merv Griffin at Cesar's Palace, Lillian glided onto the stage of the huge theater in a flowing blue dress, and accepted a standing ovation as if she had been accustomed to them all her life. Seated with her, Griffin said, "You look sensational." Without missing a beat, Lillian turned to the audience and said, "I *know* it!"[2]

More travel followed Lillian's big African trip. She went to Ireland, where she said the best thing about being there was that "I get to kiss so many men."[3] She would also travel back to Europe and even farther afield, to Egypt and Israel, and she met most of the heads of state of the day, living and deceased: she was so often sent to state funerals as representative of the Carter Administration she began to crack jokes about it. "I have a long

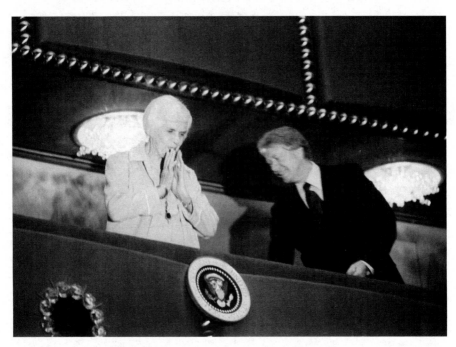

Lillian acknowledging applause at the Kennedy Center in Washington, D.C., in April 1977; President Carter leans down to pull out a chair for her (courtesy Jimmy Carter Presidential Library).

black dress and a short black dress," she quipped to a reporter, "because whenever a foreigner dies it seems like everybody's busy but me." She was on hand to greet her second pope, John Paul II, who visited the White House in 1979. His Holiness had the unique experience of watching the eighty-one year old First Mother careen toward him in high heels over a newly waxed floor. Neither, according to Jimmy Carter, was at a loss for words. "Holy Father," said Lillian, still smitten by the handsome pontiff she had "chosen," "I made this dramatic entrance just for you." Said a smiling John Paul II, "I enjoyed it very much." Lillian loved President Anwar Sadat of Egypt as much as her son did, declaring him "my favorite of all men in the world"; but it was Lillian whom Israel's Menachem Begin was first to embrace just after the signing with Sadat of the first of the peace treaties brokered by President Carter. "All the time she was sending kisses to me in the air!" a delighted Begin commented to Carter.[4]

During these years, Lillian also became a favorite "draw" for Democratic politicians campaigning for office. In September 1978 she flew to Arkansas to help out Doug Brandon in his ultimately unsuccessful race for a congressional seat, then on to Kansas to support future State Supreme Court Justice and then candidate for Fifth District Congressional seat Donald L. Allegrucci, enjoying all the while town hall meetings with Young Democrats and dinner parties at private homes and historic sites. (While in Little Rock, she telephoned Jimmy after watching him on television with Israeli Prime Minister Menachem Begin and Egyptian President Anwar Sadat. "Jimmy," she asked coyly, "is Anwar Sadat already married?") Later that month, Lillian flew to New Jersey for events benefiting the campaign of Congressman Frank Thompson, followed by a Long Island appearance for Congressman Tom Downey and another in Westchester County for Congressman Dick Ottinger. It was a heavy schedule for a woman of eight decades; that year, Lillian ultimately visited some twenty-one candidates across the country. Lillian enjoyed proving the Peace Corps adage that age was no barrier. "I hope I die with my shoes on," she told a reporter during her campaign visits. And she was having fun, as were the politicians she helped. One of those who benefited from her visit was future U.S. Senator Tom Daschle of South Dakota, then running against Republican Leo Thorsness for the First District seat. (He won by a margin of 139 votes.) Born in 1947, Daschle was a native of Aberdeen, and was just thirty-one when the eighty year old Lillian flew into town to categorically tell people: "You all should vote for this young man as your next Congressman." Daschle was flattered that the president's famous mother had made time for him. He remembers being amazed not only that she had come to South

Dakota but wanted to take part in his rigorous campaign schedule. "I had made quite a thing of going door to door," he recalls. "And here she was, in her early eighties, and she was prepared to go door to door with me. This charmed everybody, of course, but nobody as much as the media." Even the barefoot housewife surprised in her ironing was too delighted to care about the intrusion. "I knew that you were coming to town," she told a smiling Lillian, "but not that you were coming to see me." At a reception later Lillian regaled guests with remarks about how her son kept her so busy but how wonderful it was to never retire; how she couldn't abide red wine "but a little white wine isn't bad," and how she was counting the hours till the rematch between Leon Spinks and her favorite Muhammad Ali scheduled for later that month. As Daschle recalls, she made a hit everywhere they went.[5]

The sheer variety and unlikelihood of experiences Lillian had as First Mother are possibly best exemplified by her visit to Studio 54, New York City's discothèque par excellence, in December 1977.

Studio 54 had a relatively brief existence as nightclubs go. From 1977 until the 1980 arrest of founders Steve Rubell and Ian Schrager on tax evasion and conspiracy charges, it was the hub of a wildly spinning Manhattan nightlife in which a broad spectrum of partiers boogied to Donna Summer or the Village People. Movie stars and rock stars, debutantes and demi-mondes, fashion designers and politicians, princesses and publicity hounds all delighted to be seen in a club that became a cornerstone of out and proud gay culture and a locus of the drug activity that fueled the disco high. In keeping with Studio 54's permanent atmosphere of arch irony, it was India and the children's charity UNICEF which brought Lillian there for a party meant to raise funds for the latter while celebrating the sesquicentennial of the city of Jaipur. And sometime that evening the Indian Ambassador and civil rights activist Nani A. Palkhivala was scheduled to present Lillian with the Indo-American Peace and Friendship award.[6]

The Jaipur Ball, as it was called, had plenty of Indian touches. Indian musicians played authentic music in the background as a young lady wearing a sari scattered artificial rose petals over each VIP who came in the door: C.Z. Guest, Estée Lauder, Halston, Andy Warhol. The latter, who arrived with Lillian on his arm, may seem an unlikely escort. Yet Warhol, with his keen eye for life's satire, was fascinated by a woman who, had she been like most eighty-year-old ladies, would have been living out her golden years in a quiet cottage, knitting or playing solitaire rather than shaking her groove thing at America's most notorious dance club. He knew she was something different. A few months before the Jaipur Ball, Warhol wrote, he went with Steve Rubell to see Lillian at the Waldorf Hotel. A dinner had been planned for her there by United Jewish Appeal (later United Jewish Communities), a group founded in 1939 which raised and distributed funds to help Jews in Europe, Palestine and elsewhere. During the dinner, Lillian would be presented with the group's Outstanding Humanitarian of the Year award as well as an $18,000 stipend, which she gave to charity. Warhol met her in a reception room at the Waldorf before the event. "She was thrilled to see me," he wrote, and told him how much she enjoyed the photographs he had taken of her; one of these was used to create a portrait to help raise funds for Jimmy Carter's second run for president. During the dinner, Warhol sat with increasing boredom until Lillian got on stage to accept her award. She said, "I've never met so many Jews in my life!," a remark that Warhol claims went over the crowd like a shock wave. Nobody was sure just what she meant. Then the room erupted in laughter and applause—in true Miss Lillian style, the tone of serious high purpose had been breached and people could relax. "She was good," commented Warhol with rare approval.[7]

The Jaipur Ball had been pushed back to 10 p.m. to allow for private dinner parties, at one of which Lillian had been Mrs. Guest's guest of honor, but most were still late showing up at the club. In fact, by the time Lillian reached her table, Ambassador Palkhivala (who would be censured and recalled after a photograph of him helping Lillian put on a shoe was released in India)[8] had left the building, according to *New York Times* society columnist Enid Nemy, and his seat was taken by Warhol. "The crush in the reserved area was so great that, at times, it was worth their seats for any of the guests to get up and greet friends," wrote Nemy. "Mrs. Carter did so a few times and would have been chairless on her return had not Steve Rubell, the club owner, preceded her to the table. 'Mrs. Carter is returning,' he would say, fixing a no-nonsense eye on the body in the chair at the moment."[9] With Rubell watching out for her seat, Lillian was able to take to the dance floor where she took a turn or two with bearded, bespectacled party organizer George-Paul Rosell; photographs appeared a few days later showing her, wearing what Warhol might have termed "a sort-of-nightie," as he did another of her outfits, ending the dance "with a flourish."[10] Amid the goings on that evening, which besides the loud crowd and loud music included live doves fluttering about people's heads and a peacock that preened at seeing its reflection, Lillian kept her composure. "Upon being presented to couturier Halston, [Lillian] asked him if he was Italian," wrote

Earl Wilson. "He's from the Midwest," Wilson pointed out. Lillian adored Italian men—"I've never seen an ugly Italian" she told reporters on her arrival in Rome—so this may had been a case of wishful thinking.[11]

If we are to believe Steve Rubell, Lillian turned to him during the Jaipur Ball to ask "Why are all these boys dancing together? There are all these pretty girls around."[12] But Lillian was hardly ignorant of homosexuality or of the problems faced by gay people. Her son, after all, was the first United States president to deal positively with the issue of gay rights. Yet before that, Lillian was already making her opinion known on the subject. "You remember Anita Bryant?" she asked Henry Mitchell of the *Washington Post*. "I was crazy about her—the sweetest little singer." But when she heard Bryant's anti-gay crusade speeches, Lillian said, "I feel absolute disgust for her." Mitchell had suggested that perhaps Lillian should tell Bryant to mind her own business. "Oh, I did," she said.[13] In 1979, Lillian and California Governor Edmund G. Brown took part in a dinner to raise money for the Gay Community Services Center in Los Angeles. Interviewed at the Beverly Wilshire Hotel, Lillian responded to all the questions the best way she knew how, by being maddeningly oblique. On the eve of the AIDS pandemic, when every dollar would soon count very much indeed, Lillian was asked if it embarrassed her to raise funds for the gay community at the dinner. Lillian replied, "No, not at all. Is that what it is?" Which about sums up her scorn for nosy reporters and for those who assumed she was too old or protected to know the facts of life.[14]

Nor had she been in the dark regarding the undercurrent of illicit substances flowing through the club that night of the Jaipur Ball. Village People member Randy Jones was later to insist that he had witnessed a joint being handed around at Studio 54, which happened to end up in Lillian's hand. "She looked horrified," he recalled. "She didn't take a puff, but she handed it to me very expertly." Lillian was clearly "horrified" more by the possibility that even handling a joint would make its way into the press and harm her son than she was about the joint itself; her passing it along showed that while she had to be prudent for herself she did not judge others.[15] In any case, her feelings about her night at Studio 54 were unambivalent. "I'm not sure if it was heaven or hell," she said. "But it was wonderful."[16]

It wasn't that Lillian didn't also find a piece of heaven back home in Plains, or rather, at her Pond House. She just had to increasingly hide out to find it.

In Plains itself, she told Jimmy, she felt like she was a prisoner because of tourists crowding the streets, even trying to peek in the windows of her red brick house to watch her watching her soap operas. "I haven't been downtown since December," she complained to a reporter in May 1977. "People swarm around me and crush me.... I really don't get any privacy, and I don't get to go out much." Being the mother of the president was, in her words, "a mixed blessing."[17]

Many of these people gravitated to Lillian not just because she was, as she once put it, the next best thing to meeting her son, but also because she was so loved and admired and so certain to say something unexpected and possibly shocking. But she was getting tired of the performance. Jimmy wrote that toward the end of his term, his mother shifted more and more of her belongings out of town and into the Pond House.[18] It was there that she had the quiet she desired and needed in order to deal with correspondence befitting a movie star, with Jan Williams as her secretary.

Williams had been Amy Carter's teacher, presiding over a class of fourth graders one of whom had two Secret Service men standing nearby at all times. This led to Williams looking after Amy from time to time and eventually to answering mail for her. In those pre-computer days, Williams had to type every reply on an electronic typewriter. "For every letter Amy received, her father told me, 'We must respond, because we can always put at the end of the letter, Please ask your mom and dad to vote for my daddy,'" Williams recalls. More important than soliciting votes, she says, was making sure children who wrote to Amy knew that in many respects her life was not all that different from theirs—that she had favorite television shows, had a certain time by which she had to go to bed, and that standards applied to any other child were rigorously applied to her.[19]

"During the presidential campaign, we began to notice that Miss Lillian was getting a lot of mail," Williams says, "not unlike what Amy received—people asking about her son and what kind of man he was and about Miss Lillian's life. Because of my closeness to Amy, Miss Lillian said she'd like for me to write *her* letters. So after teaching all day, one afternoon I would spend reading letters that came to an older woman and composing responses as if I was her. Then the next day I might be the eight year old girl and have to compose letters answering questions sent to Amy." The letters Lillian received covered a wide range of topics and requests, from the serious—as when the mother of Soviet *refusnik* Anatoly Scharansky pleaded for her help in getting her son out of a Siberian labor camp—to dubious appeals from pseudo-religious groups in India and the United States. The more complicated letters were answered by White House staff after appropriate review, but straightforward missives to grandmother and granddaughter were within Williams' purview. Both Amy and Lillian always signed their own letters, a chore of which Amy tired quickly enough, given her age. Lillian, on the other hand, was happy to autograph into infinity. "Some days I would take Miss Lillian twenty-five or thirty letters, which was really a lot," says Williams, "and yet she would be furious with me that I didn't bring her more! And then the next day, when I might bring only fifteen, she wouldn't say a word. With Miss Lillian, that's the way it was—whichever way the wind blew."[20]

Williams remembers vividly the day a letter arrived from one correspondent, offering more than just abstract admiration. "They wanted to give Miss Lillian a poodle," recalls Williams. "I said, 'Miss Lillian, I'm going to send in regrets about this poodle.' She said, 'Oh, no—I would like a dog!' I said, 'Miss Lillian, it might make you trip and fall, or what about when you go off on these trips? I'll have to find somebody to take care of it.' She looked at me then as if to say, 'Why are you asking? *You're* going to be doing it.'" Ultimately Williams couldn't win out on that one. "So we got the poodle. When it came it might have been six to eight inches tall—a cute little chocolate-colored poodle. Miss Lillian named him Periwinkle (Perry for short). But then Perry began to grow. After a while, Perry was the size of a small goat. And he kept getting bigger. Soon he was a real handful. He was not obedient, and kind of did whatever *he* wanted to do."[21] As a press report noted, "Mrs. Carter's brown poodle continued to cavort among the many tourists who daily visit the Plains railroad depot, once the Carter campaign headquarters where Miss Lillian used to sit in a rocking chair and greet all comers."[22] That Lillian was aware that Perry was a problem is clear from a remark she made to Jimmy around this time. "My dog is now in obedience school," she said, by way of citing why she needed to be in Plains, "and his time is up. He's already smarter than I am."[23] In an interview, she introduced Perry to the reporter as the dog was put through his paces on her lawn, pointing out that while training was expensive, it was "worth every penny." Though her poodle was smart, he wasn't smart enough to spell, she said, "but I couldn't s-t-a-n-d poodles until I got this one."[24]

She loved him, but Perry eventually got too smart, and one day Lillian summoned Jan. "I think we're going to have to find a home for Perry," she announced. "You may take him this afternoon." Williams replied, "Now, ma'am, I didn't want him when he was little; I don't want him now," but there was no arguing with Miss Lillian.[25]

When the coast was clear, Lillian still went out from time to time. Surrounded by security, she wasn't so inconvenienced by tourists that she couldn't venture to Columbus to the wrestling matches, where she enjoyed her favorite performer, John Walker, a.k.a. Mr. Wrestling II, in action. After one of these matches, Lillian extended an invitation to Walker to come visit her at her home, "because she wanted to have a personal interview with me," Walker recalls. Reporter Richard Hyatt was with Walker for the drive down to Plains. "We went in the oversize Lincoln of Fred Ward, the wrestling promoter," says Hyatt. "He called John 'Two.' He said, 'Two, I wish you would drive this thing; I don't drive the highways much anymore.' So here we were driving along with Wrestling II at the wheel, in his mask, and as we got to Plains we started worrying what the Secret Service would think of that."[26] Walker remembers his apprehension vividly. "I never took the mask off, because I knew there would be a lot of people there who went to the matches in Columbus, and they'd be wanting to see what I looked like without it," he says. Once they arrived in Plains, "oh gosh, there were Secret Service men, State Patrol, everything else, all over the yard," Walker remembers.[27]

Walker was met at the door by Lillian, who waved at him as he came up the driveway. "Miss Lillian was so vain," recalls Hyatt, "she didn't want anyone to see her. She wasn't well and not looking her best."[28] One of Lillian's sisters was there also. As Walker recalls, Lillian "told her sister that she did not want to be disturbed. I thought that was cute." Everyone else had to wait outside.[29]

"So we went into a room, closed the door, sat down, and chatted," says Walker. "We must have talked for at least two and a half hours, just about all kinds of different things. When it was all over, the one thing that stood out to my mind was that she never came across with any sarcastic questions"—questions, that is, about wrestling. None of the Carters or friends of Lillian who attended matches with her ever believed what they were seeing was real. But Lillian respected the performance aspect of professional wrestling, and anyone Lillian admired she took very seriously. "She finally did ask me, though, 'Are you good-looking?'" Walker remembers with amusement. "She didn't ask me to take my mask off—in fact, I was really amazed she didn't ask that—she just wanted to know a bit about what I was like underneath. So I said, 'Well, my *wife* thinks I am.' How she laughed! She got the biggest kick out of that."[30] Hyatt remembers that despite Lillian's vanity, Fred Ward's granddaughter was able to take a photograph of her with Walker. Hyatt remembers this photograph showing up later in a wrestling magazine. "And then it appeared on Saturday Night Live," he recalls. "Jane Curtin gave the Weekend Update, saying something like 'The White House is shocked and concerned to hear that Miss Lillian

Carter will marry heavyweight wrestler Mr. Wrestling II...."[31] The transcript for that segment has Lillian saying, "I beat him, two out of three falls, and he proposed on the spot."[32]

Walker remembers that a week or so later, he received a call from Lillian. "She asked me if I would mind making a personal appearance at a Special Olympics event in Plains," he says. He was delighted to do so, as much to meet the kids as to see Lillian again. A friend who owned a private plane flew Walker down to Plains, where Lillian had arranged for him to be brought to the ballpark where so many softball games had been played during the presidential campaign. "The kids gave me a wonderful welcome," says Walker, who is still so much in demand that at his recent induction into the Professional Wrestling Hall of Fame in New York State, he had lines of autograph seekers and well-wishers filing past him all evening. "They just hollered and screamed," he remembers. "I spent the whole time with Lillian and just loved it."[33]

"She was the best woman in the world," says Walker. "I have more respect for her than I do anybody."[34]

One of the last references to Lillian's poodle came in the middle of an article about her campaigning for Jimmy, who was running for another four years as president.

Lillian was in Miami at the end of August 1979. When asked if she had ever been there, she answered that she had indeed, "dozens of times," adding, "I hate it. I don't consider it a part of the United States. It's such a hodge-podge, and so crowded." Questioned as to why she bothered to come there at all, she replied drily, "To let everybody see me and see how sweet I am." She went, she said, because Jimmy asked her to do so, though of course she would rather be home at the Pond House with Perry.[35] Less than three months later, on November 2, 1979, the United States Embassy in Teheran was overtaken by Islamist militants, and it was the beginning of the end of the Carter administration and the start of a new era in radical terrorism.

By any measure, the years 1979–1980 were *anni horribili* for President Jimmy Carter. Looking back at them is not unlike reviewing the case records of a hopelessly ill patient who nonetheless refuses to give up, even when all signs are that the end is near. The primary malady was the Iranian hostage crisis, but there had been an underlying condition, like a low-grade yet incrementally damaging fever. There was the energy crisis, with cars lined up at gas stations across the nation and Carter's under-appreciated effort to convince Americans to use less energy parodied by the media and

in people's living rooms. There was Carter's controversial decision to allow
the Shah of Iran to undergo medical treatment in the United States after
he had been deposed in 1979. The Shah's stay was brief—between October
and December—but by the time he was on his way again revolutionaries
had kidnapped American diplomatic staff in Teheran and were parading
them before the cameras of the world. The administration's rescue mission
failed miserably. Along with these conditions came allegations of Billy
Carter's improper dealings with Libya, accusations which were never
proved but which set up in Billy's life a tragic momentum toward self-
destruction. Within Jimmy and Rosalynn's immediate family, the estrange-
ment and divorce of son Chip and wife Caron seemed to mirror the split
occurring within the Democratic party, helping smooth the path for Ronald
Reagan's landslide win in 1980. Even Lillian was not immune to this flood
of ill luck. While getting up to turn on her television in autumn 1980, she
tripped over a rug and broke her right hip.[36] Carter flew down from Washington to be with his mother at Sumter County Hospital, where he stayed
the better part of an hour.[37]

This accident was a huge letdown for Lillian, because she had been
very involved in the 1980 campaign. As before, she and Rosalynn went to
New Hampshire, which had been such a lucky state for Carter in 1976.
And in August, Lillian again became a fixture at the Democratic National
Convention, this time in New York City. A young journalism graduate
named Steven Hunsicker had been given permission by the radio station
where he worked to cover the convention. He and the reporter who accompanied him had their hands full. "We split our time," Hunsicker recalls,
"either in the media center, on the convention floor, and covering caucuses."
One day he was especially busy. "I was running late, to cover a caucus meeting of the West Virginia delegation"—West Virginia University was his
alma mater. He sprinted for an open elevator, but as he got in and the doors
were sliding shut a man in a suit thrust his hand between to hold them
open. "I'm about ready to tell him to take another elevator," he remembers,
"when in walked Lillian Carter." Hunsicker had been fascinated by Lillian
since his teens, when he heard a report on television about her stint in the
Peace Corps. "My parents had to explain what the Peace Corps was," he
says. "I thought it would be a great thing to volunteer one day." Standing
in the elevator with this legend, Hunsicker was speechless, but Lillian soon
took care of that. "She broke the ice," he says. "She picked up the Secret
Service credential I was wearing, looked at it, looked at me, and said, 'You
look really cute in your picture, Steve,' reading my name off the credential."
It turned out Lillian was also headed for the West Virginia caucus meeting,

and en route she asked Hunsicker many questions—where he worked, what he wanted to do. "I asked if I could interview her," he recalls. "She said sure." Lillian was there to whip up the West Virginia caucus, and before sitting down with Hunsicker she "flashed her big smile at everyone," but her attention was reserved all for him. Though his tape recorder battery maddeningly failed and he captured no more than "one usable sound bite," Hunsicker remembers more of a conversation than questions and answers, and what a thrill it seemed for Lillian when he told her that he had been born in Georgia. "Surprisingly, I don't think we talked about the Peace Corps that day," he says. Yet he would one day work for the Peace Corps, telling the story of Lillian's service in India to prospective volunteers. As with so many who became involved in the organization, Lillian had shown Hunsicker the way: after a broadcasting career of over two decades, he, too, would become a Peace Corps Volunteer (in the Kingdom of Tonga). And as with so many who knew Lillian, though his time with her was brief, "it was memorable not just because of who she was," he says, "but because of *how* she was."[38]

Alongside domestic politics, Lillian involved herself, briefly, in inter-

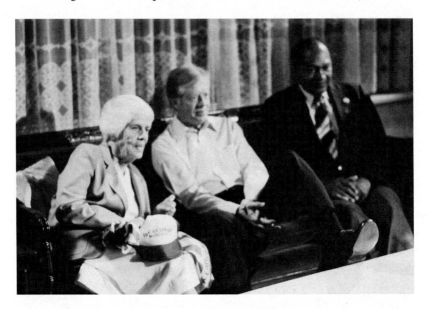

Lillian with son Jimmy Carter and Los Angeles Mayor Thomas Bradley, watching the Democratic National Convention in August 1980. When her son lost the election to Gerald R. Ford, Lillian was relieved. "I wanted [Jimmy] out—my whole family had been attacked and split wide open from Jimmy being president" (courtesy Jimmy Carter Presidential Library).

national diplomacy. "Early in December," wrote Jimmy Carter, "I was surprised to receive a phone call from Muhammad Ali, who was in Las Vegas with Mama." Ali was as much a fan of Lillian's as she was of him; in 1978 he'd given her a pair of boxing gloves autographed with a sweet message: "To Miss Lillian Carter, Service to others is the rent your son pays for his room here on earth, Love always, Muhammad Ali."[39] Lillian had told Ali that if a prominent Muslim like himself would reach out to the Ayatollah Khomeini, there might be a way to negotiate the American hostages back home. Carter took the offer seriously. "I had some of our national security officials talk to [Ali]," he wrote. But Ali's attempts to open dialogue with the Iranian regime went nowhere.[40] It probably didn't help that when Lillian spoke to a men's club in Bow, New Hampshire a few weeks after the hostage crisis began, she said, "If I had a million dollars to spare, I'd look for someone to kill [the Ayatollah]." According to a press report, she received a standing ovation for this comment, and one man shouted out that "if we were voting for the mother of the president, I know who'd win." Damage control had to go into overdrive to dampen the fallout. Lillian didn't shrink from revisiting the subject. As she told Justine De Lacey of the *International Herald Tribune*, "I'm sure I said what the whole world felt."[41]

That was all far away from the First Mother now confined to Sumter County Hospital. Following an operation to repair her hip, Lillian had to be kept there for thirty-five days, and from her bed would have seen on her television not just how poorly the Carter campaign was faring but all the publicity around Billy's Libya problem, the continued hostage drama in Iran, and the media circus that followed her family around like biting clouds of no-see-ums.

The morning of the election, which was also the first anniversary of the storming of the United States Embassy in Teheran, Lillian was still in Sumter County Hospital when Jimmy came to visit her. Jimmy told her frankly that he believed he was going to lose this election. It would have been well within reason for any mother to burst into tears at this bleak predicament, especially after the golden beginning of 1976. Yet Lillian was openly relieved. "Good!" she told him. She later said, "I wanted [Jimmy] out—my whole family had been attacked and split wide open from Jimmy being president."[42] To a reporter, she said, "I am a small town person. I keep the home fires burning. This is where I am happiest. And this is where I find peace—peace of mind and peace of body." She just wanted all her loved ones to come home.[43]

Lillian didn't return to the Pond House until April 1981, after she had convalesced at Wise Sanitarium (now the Lillian G. Carter Nursing Center). She was brought home on condition that she permit the company of a nurse, who would help her continue with therapy. And she promised to fish only when seated in a chair on her pier. Despite these restrictions, she was in seventh heaven. Having run a nursing home herself, she dreaded the thought of ever being in one and she behaved herself, for the most part. "We'd drive up and she'd be sitting there in her chair and would turn around to see who it was, because she had been reading," says Kim Carter Fuller. "It was often one of those Harlequin romances, and she didn't want just anybody to know that she read that kind of book. She would hide it and then after seeing it was us, pull it back out again."[44]

With Jimmy and Rosalynn living in Plains again, busy putting their lives financial and spiritual back together, Lillian regained some of her former energy. In August 1981, she helped her son and daughter-in-law host a visit at their Plains home from Egyptian President Anwar Sadat and his wife Jehan. Carter gave them a laurel wreath sculpted out of glass by Georgia artist Hans Frabel. Sadat and Carter discussed the need to carry out the Camp David pledges to the letter, and they also enjoyed what was described as a "delightful family visit."[45] A month later, Israeli Prime Minister Menachem Begin arrived in Plains for a visit, and Lillian met again the man at whom she had sent air kisses at the Camp David treaty signing ceremony of a few years earlier.[46]

In June, just two months after returning home, Lillian had a routine medical examination during which she was found to have a malignant tumor in her left breast. She underwent a modified radical mastectomy and her personal physician issued a statement of cautious optimism.[47]

Soon after, the family's attention was diverted from Lillian's health to that of Ruth Carter Stapleton. In April 1983, Ruth was diagnosed with terminal cancer of the pancreas—the same disease that had taken Earl Carter in 1953. Her son, Dr. Scott Stapleton, an ophthalmologist, urged his mother to seek orthodox treatment, but Ruth would have none of it. "My whole life has been geared to this kind of thing," she told the press. "I worked twenty years in healing, and I have seen so many miracles." She pursued a course of "treatments" involving exercises, diet and prayer.[48] Jimmy Carter indicates that his sister also tried chemotherapy. He and Rosalynn took Lillian along on their trips to visit Ruth in Fayetteville, North Carolina. "We had to acknowledge Ruth's obvious lack of progress," wrote Carter. A photograph taken on one of these trips of Ruth embracing Lillian shows how wasted Ruth's body was, even as the love between mother and daughter glows like the sunshine in their hair.[49]

Lillian herself was in the hospital when Ruth passed away on September 26, 1983. That summer, Lillian had told Jimmy that she had discovered a lump in her right breast. Tests were run. "Within a few days," wrote Carter, "we learned that it was malignant and had seriously metastasized, even to her pancreas." The family kept her at her beloved Pond House as long as possible, but had to admit her to hospital care in Americus when her condition worsened. The Carters were surprised at how accepting she was of the prognosis, not unlike her reaction to the news that her son had lost the election. She was, says Carter, more focused on settling her family's fears than making a big show of her own.[50]

Kim Carter Fuller remembers that when Ruth died, her mother Sybil stayed at the hospital with Lillian while Fuller and the rest of the family went to the funeral. "Grandmama called me on the phone," recalls Fuller, "and she said, 'Now when you get home you come up here and tell me what it was like.' So I went over to Americus to describe the funeral for her. She wanted the information first hand—she didn't want to just read about it." Ruth had always been Earl Carter's special darling, and she was special to Lillian as well. The pain of losing Earl returned with the loss of Ruth. "She told me, after Aunt Ruth died, that the most awful thing for a mother was for a child to die before she did," says Kim Carter Fuller. "She said that after Granddaddy died, she thought she would never hurt that way again. But with Aunt Ruth's death, it was ten times worse." Fuller thinks that Ruth's death dealt her grandmother a blow that she didn't have the will to resist. "I think she just gave up," she says. "I think the grief was just too much for her." Lillian asked that her grandchildren be brought to her, one at a time, to see her, then told Billy that she did not want them to see her again before she died. All obeyed except Fuller. "I stayed in the waiting room," she says. "I couldn't leave."[51]

Lillian Gordy Carter died in Americus on October 30, surrounded by family, a little over a month after the death of her daughter Ruth. She was eighty-five years old.

"Her body was brought to the funeral home," recalls Fuller, and was dressed in her favorite blue evening gown. "Aunt Gogo [Gloria] told me that Grandmama had left instructions that I was to do her makeup." Fuller went to the funeral home with her father, Billy. "I will never forget walking in with him," she says. "I had her lipstick and her powder—she didn't wear much makeup at all—and Daddy said, 'She looks just like she did when we were children.' Daddy and I brushed her hair."[52]

As Fuller and her father started to leave, Billy turned around. "He said, 'She's just too pretty—we can't just leave her here,'" remembers Fuller. "So we did something that not many folks in Plains did then. We had her body brought home, to the Pond House, and placed on her bed. And Daddy sat up with her all night, while people came through during the night to talk to her." Rick Hutto arrived next morning to be greeted on the Pond House driveway by Emily Dolvin. "I went up and gave her a big kiss," he recalls, "and she asked, 'Have you seen Lillian?' I told her I hadn't had time to stop at the funeral home, and had been told to come straight to the Pond House. She said, 'No, honey, she's in here! Come on, let me take you.'" In the living room, Hutto found a crowd of mourners combined of old family friends and relatives and former Carter administration staff like Bert Lance. There was even a Saudi prince.[53] The mood was one of lightness, not grief. Though devastated and haggard after a sleepless night, Billy still had a spark of humor that echoed his mother's. "When somebody asked Daddy what it was like in Grandmama's bedroom that night," recalls Fuller, "he said, 'Well, Mama never said a word!'"[54]

Lillian had left a detailed list of who she wanted invited to her funeral and who was to make themselves scarce. "She had people she wanted there," says Fuller, "and people she did not!" One of them, a man with whom Lillian had had a falling out, had originally been deleted from the list of invitees, but when they made up she had added him back in. In all, some three hundred people attended the funeral in early November. She was interred next to Earl Carter in the family plot in Lebanon Cemetery, located on a rise of red earth among the pines trees outside Plains. The ceremony lasted just a few minutes, per Lillian's specific request.[55]

One neighbor was heard to remark afterward that "that's what she wanted, short and simple." Another quipped, "And she usually got her way."[56]

Epilogue

One golden October afternoon very near the twenty-seventh anniversary of Lillian Carter's death, I sat in the living room of the Pond House with her granddaughter, Kim Carter Fuller.

After all the to-do of getting there, which involved entering a restricted area and fetching a key from Secret Service, the peace was profound.

We walked up the driveway that meanders among Georgia pines, swatting at gnats we could actually hear. The trees stand very close to the driveway's edge, making me wonder how Lillian maneuvered her car through them without incident. As she once told a television talk show host, "I've never hit a tree, but I've been *exposed*." Luckily, her family intervened before exposure developed into a dented fender or worse. "They put down asphalt for Grandmama after they took away her driving privileges," Fuller told me. "It was so she could keep driving her car a little around the paved area."[1] It was strangely moving to envision the small, white-haired old lady, slowly taking her vehicle up and down the driveway—she who had traveled so far, who loved nothing so much as a good-looking car. That isn't to say, though, that she really yearned to go anywhere anymore. Being here, I could see why. Just as they did the day Orde Coombs came to interview her, Lillian's squirrels scrambled up and down the trees; over her pond's jade surface a snowy egret glided, a Chinese scroll painting in the middle of southwest Georgia. Out here in the woods, on this low rise, even the presence of fields buzzing at harvest time was screened out along with the rest of the noisy world.

Once in the Pond House itself, I roamed at Fuller's urging. Everywhere there were books—Emil Ludwig's *The Nile*, Thomas Costain's *The Conquering Family*, even a worn New Testament given to Billy Carter as a boy by his cousin, "Tody," the William Spann of troubled future decades.

There were African and Indian artifacts, a zebra rug and objects which, if they were not all Lillian's own, did reflect her eclectic decorating style, in which she made her living room a kind of gallery for the exotic gifts presented to her on her travels.

There was also a fair representation of modern art. On one wall hung LeRoy Neiman's pencil sketch of Lillian, created on her birthday in August 1980 as she sat in her balcony at the Democratic National Convention. Lillian's strong profile is surrounded by the ephemera of political rallies— placards shouting Jimmy Carter's virtues, clouds of faded red and blue balloons. Neiman's Lillian looks obdurate, determined to last out the evening. Yet there is a sense, too, that she would far rather be at the Pond House, away from balloons and baloney. Jimmy lost the election and Lillian got her wish: she won back her family.

Much of Lillian's original furniture is still in the house. In the front windows still stand the table, lamp, chair and television pictured in dozens of newspaper and magazine features. And in the little back bedroom is the small bed where Billy had her body placed the night before the funeral, where he sat with her, talking against the darkness and the silence.

For an hour, Fuller and I sat in Lillian's living room. We conversed on a range of pressing subjects so near to Lillian's heart it would not have surprised either of us had she suddenly entered the room and joined in: bullying in schools, race relations, broken families, and the unconditional love we learned from our grandmothers, who both insisted it was the panacea for most any hurt.

And sometimes we just sat there without speaking, absorbing the house's glow. In all my study of books and articles, oral histories and videotapes and interviews with those who knew Lillian Carter personally, I had never touched on the key to who she really was, as person and personality, until that autumn afternoon in the Pond House, the pines looking in at us through the high windows, the squirrels scooting up and down.

Lillian Carter loved her family, but she didn't really belong to it alone, neither as a young wife and mother nor as an elder matriarch and grandmother. She belonged, and still belongs, not to the Carters or Gordys, nor to the United States of America, or to India, but to the world at large. Its pains and problems were as much hers to soothe and solve as those of her husband and children, and she did what she could to solve them.

"She died and left us all behind," wrote Jimmy Carter in a poem titled simply, "Miss Lillian." "What will we do now?"[2] Lillian would have had a simple answer. Just keep caring, keep soothing, and most of all, keep *loving*.

Notes

Preface

1. Nina Strawser, "A Tribute to My Era," 1970, unpublished manuscript, Nina Strawser Papers.

2. Nina Strawser, "A Prescription for Peace," 1967, unpublished manuscript, Nina Strawser Papers.

3. Lillian Carter with Gloria Carter Spann, *Away from Home* (New York: Simon & Schuster, 1977), p. 153. Hereafter *AFM*.

4. Jimmy Carter to author, March 2011.

5. Jimmy Carter to author, October 2012.

Chapter 1

1. Orde Coombs, "The Hand That Rocked Carter's Cradle," *New York Magazine*, June 14, 1976, p. 40.

2. Jimmy Carter, *A Remarkable Mother* (New York: Simon & Schuster, 2008), p. 153. Hereafter *ARM*.

3. David Alsobrook to author, June 2011.

4. Ibid.

5. Coombs, p. 41.

6. David Alsobrook Oral History Interview with Lillian Carter, Sept. 26, 1978.

7. Ibid.

8. Ibid.

9. Ibid.

10. Jimmy Carter gubernatorial inauguration speech, Jan. 12, 1971; JC "on the impact of religion and tradition on the lives of women and girls," video on Elders.org and uploaded to YouTube June 26, 2009: http://

www.youtube.com/watch?v=q-JcpNBiRcM&noredirect=1 (link active as of Apr. 19, 2014).

11. David Alsobrook Oral History Interview with Lillian Carter, Sept. 26, 1978.

12. Ibid.

13. David Alsobrook Oral History Interview with Emily Gordy Dolvin, June 28, 1979.

14. Kenneth H. Thomas, Jr., *Georgia Life*, Winter 1976, pp. 40–46 and Spring 1980, pp. 40–43 (hereafter KHT); Gary Boyd Roberts, *Ancestors of American Presidents* (Boston: New England Historic Genealogical Society, 2009), pp. 167–174. According to Nelson George, *Where Did Our Love Go? The Rise & Fall of the Motown Sound* (Sydney: Omnibus Press, 1987), pp. 1–2, and Jeff Carter, *Ancestors of Jimmy and Rosalynn Carter* (Jefferson, NC: McFarland, 2012), p. 94, James Thomas Gordy fathered a son by a slave named Esther Johnson. Their child, Berry Gordy, was born in 1854, and was the grandson of Motown founder Berry Gordy.

15. Jimmy Carter, *An Hour Before Daylight: Memories of a Rural Boyhood* (New York: Simon & Schuster, 2001), pp. 241–244 (hereafter *AHBD*); KHT, Winter 1976, pp. 40–46 and Spring 1980, pp. 40–43.

16. *AHBD*, pp. 241–244; KHT, Winter 1976, pp. 40–46 and Spring 1980, pp. 40–43.

17. KHT, Winter 1976, pp. 40–46 and Spring 1980, pp. 40–43; Thomas told the author (Apr. 9, 2011) he heard Lillian deny to a reporter that her ancestors had owned

slaves; Jimmy Carter did so himself early in his campaign but subsequently acknowledged the truth; see James Wooten, *Dasher: The Roots and Raising of Jimmy Carter* (New York: Simon & Schuster, 1978), p. 63.

18. KHT, Spring 1980, p. 43.

19. David Alsobrook Oral History Interview with Elizabeth Gordy Braunstein, Nov. 14, 1979.

20. David Alsobrook Oral History Interview with Emily Gordy Dolvin, June 28, 1979.

21. Marie Allen Oral History Interview with Fanny Surasky Gordy, Feb. 11, 1980.

22. "Mr. D.C. Gordy Ends His Life; Sad Death of a Prominent Citizen of Chattahoochee," *Columbus Daily Enquirer*, Nov. 13, 1902.

23. Beth Tartan and Rudy Hayes, *Miss Lillian and Friends: The Plains, Georgia Family Philosophy and Recipe Book* (New York: Signet, 1977), p. 3. Hereafter *ML&F*.

24. David Alsobrook Oral History Interview with Emily Gordy Dolvin, June 28, 1979. Jimmy Carter wrote me that "Tom Watson was in the U.S. Congress from 1891–1893 and *was* a State Senator from 1921 until his death. Jim Jack gave Tom Watson the idea for RFD."

25. David Alsobrook Oral History Interview with Elizabeth Gordy Braunstein, Nov. 14, 1979.

26. David Alsobrook Oral History Interview with Lillian Carter, Sept. 26, 1978.

27. Marie Allen Oral History Interview with Fanny Surasky Gordy, Feb. 11, 1980.

28. David Alsobrook Oral History Interview with Lillian Carter, Sept. 26, 1978; David Alsobrook Oral History Interview with Elizabeth Gordy Braunstein, Nov. 14, 1979. Jimmy Carter wrote me that "Daddy didn't plow (I did) but he did all other jobs on the farm."

29. David Alsobrook Oral History Interview with Lillian Carter, Sept. 26, 1978.

30. *ARM*, p. 20.

31. David Alsobrook Oral History Interview with Elizabeth Gordy Braunstein, Nov. 14, 1979.

32. *ARM*, p. 12.

33. Ibid., p. 8.

34. David Alsobrook Oral History Interview with Emily Gordy Dolvin, June 28, 1979.

35. Ibid.

36. Wooten, p. 71.

37. David Alsobrook Oral History Interview with Lillian Carter, Sept. 26, 1978.

38. *ARM*, p. 2.

39. Letter of Jan. 6, 1916, from Tom Watson to James Jackson Gordy, University of North Carolina Library.

40. Tad Brown of the Watson-Brown Foundation, email to author, Mar. 14, 2011.

41. David Alsobrook Oral History Interview with Lillian Carter, Sept. 26, 1978. Lillian described her three years at the Richland post office in *Postal Life*, March/April 1977, "Miss Lillian and Miss Allie Talk Post Office."

42. Ibid. The 1900 United States Census for Richland, Georgia, shows the Gordys as one of the few white families on their road, but this should not be taken as indicating that they lived in a predominantly black neighborhood. As Kenneth H. Thomas, Jr., explains, in most circumstances these black families lived near white ones because they worked for them, or because they rented property from them, which would speak to their large numbers. However, it is significant that in the 1930 Census, as Mrs. James Earl Carter, Lillian was again living surrounded by black families—her husband's tenant farmers.

43. *ARM*, p. 3.

44. Stephen G.N. Tuck, *Beyond Atlanta: The Struggle for Racial Equality in Georgia, 1940–1980* (Athens: University of Georgia Press, 2003), pp. 19–25.

45. David Alsobrook Oral History Interview with Lillian Carter, Sept. 26, 1978.

46. Coombs, p. 42.

Chapter 2

1. David Alsobrook Oral History Interview with Lillian Carter, Sept. 26, 1978.

2. Ibid.

3. Alan Anderson, *Remembering Americus: Essays on Southern Life* (Charleston: History Press, 2006), pp. 58–60.

4. David Alsobrook Oral History Interview with Lillian Carter, Sept. 26, 1978.

5. *AHBD*, p. 14.

6. *ARM*, p. 60.

7. Ibid., p. 62.

8. David Alsobrook Oral History Interview with Lillian Carter, Sept. 26, 1978.

9. Ibid.

10. Ibid.

11. *ARM*, p. 55.

12. Shamim M. Baker, Otis W. Brawley, and Leonard S. Marks, "Effects of Untreated Syphilis in the Negro Male, 1932 to 1972: A Closure Comes to the Tuskegee Study, 2004," *Urology* 65(6), 2005.

13. W.E.B. Du Bois, *The Souls of Black Folk* (New York: Barnes and Noble Classics, 2003), p. 16.

14. *ARM*, p. 55.

15. Tuck, p. 15.

16. *AHBD*, p. 83; *ARM*, pp. 57–59.

17. David Alsobrook Oral History Interview with Lillian Carter, Sept. 26, 1978.

18. *ARM*, p. 16.

19. David Alsobrook Oral History Interview with Lillian Carter, Sept. 26, 1978.

20. Ibid.

21. Douglas Brinkley, "A Time for Reckoning: Jimmy Carter and the Cult of Kinfolk," *Presidential Studies Quarterly* 29 (1999): 778–798.

22. David Alsobrook Oral History Interview with Lillian Carter, Sept. 26, 1978.

23. *ARM*, pp. 19–20; David Alsobrook Oral History Interview with Lillian Carter, Sept. 26, 1978,

24. Kim Carter Fuller email to author, June 2011,

25. *ML&F*, pp. 12–13; *ARM*, p. 41; Shakespeare, *The Merchant of Venice*, Act 1, Scene 4.

26. Richard Halliburton, *The Royal Road to Romance* (Palo Alto: Travelers Tales Classics, Publishers Groups West, 2000), pp. 3–4.

27. *AHBD*, pp.136–137; Doug Wead, *The Raising of a President: The Mothers and Fathers of Our Nation's Leaders* (New York: Atria, 2005), pp. 402–403.

28. David Alsobrook Oral History Interview with Lillian Carter, Sept. 26, 1978.

29. Ibid.; *ARM*, pp. 21–22.

30. David Alsobrook Oral History Interview with Lillian Carter, Sept. 26, 1978.

31. Ibid.

32. *ARM*, p. 40.

33. David Alsobrook Oral History Interview with Emily Gordy Dolvin, June 28, 1979.

34. David Alsobrook Oral History Interview with Lillian Carter, Sept. 26, 1978.

35. Ibid.

36. Ibid.

37. *ARM*, p. 20.

38. Ibid., p. 25.

39. *ML&F*, p. 8.

Chapter 3

1. *ARM*, p. 22.

2. Ibid.

3. Ibid.

4. David Alsobrook Oral History Interview with Lillian Carter, Sept. 26, 1978.

5. *ARM*, pp. 22–23.

6. David Alsobrook Oral History Interview with Lillian Carter, Sept. 26, 1978.

7. *AHBD*, pp. 35–36.

8. Ibid., p. 16.

9. The Arts & Crafts Society, "Sears, Roebuck Houses Offered between 1908 and 1940," http://www.arts-crafts.com/archive/sears-roebuck.shtml.

10. Ruth Carter Stapleton, *Brother Billy* (New York: HarperCollins, 1978), p. 9; *The Mike Douglas Show*, WCHA # C-14, 13 December 1976/1000, CBS, "Mike Douglas Show with Lillian and Amy Carter in Plains: A Tour Through Plains," Jimmy Carter Library.

11. *ARM*, p. 26.

12. David Alsobrook Oral History Interview with Lillian Carter, Sept. 26, 1978.

13. Lillian Carter, *Guideposts*, pp. 2–4.

14. David Alsobrook Oral History Interview with Lillian Carter, Sept. 26, 1978

15. *AHBD*, pp. 22–23.

16. David Alsobrook Oral History Interview with Lillian Carter, Sept. 26, 1978.

17. Coombs, p. 42.

18. Dallas Lee, *The Cotton Patch Evidence: The Story of Clarence Jordan and Koinonia Farm Experiment* (New York: Harper & Row, 1971), p. 48.

19. *AHBD*, p. 66; Jimmy Carter to author, July 2012.

20. *AHBD*, p. 53.

21. David Alsobrook Oral History Interview with Lillian Carter, Sept. 26, 1978

22. *ARM*, p. 54.

23. Ibid., pp. 46–47.

24. David Alsobrook Oral History Interview with Lillian Carter, Sept. 26, 1978.

25. *ARM*, pp. 53–54.

26. Marie B. Allen Oral History Interview with Rachel Clark, Nov. 9, 1978.

27. *ARM*, pp. 63–64.

28. *AHBD*, p. 61.

29. Ibid., pp. 59–60.

30. Jimmy Carter, *Always a Reckoning and Other Poems* (New York: Random House, 1995), p. 19.

31. *ARM*, p. 64.

32. Coombs, p. 40.

33. David Alsobrook Oral History Interview with Lillian Carter, Sept. 26, 1978.

34. Howard Pousner, *The Atlanta Journal-Constitution*, Mar. 8, 2011.

35. *AHBD*, p. 75.

36. Stapleton, p. 43.

37. *AHBD*, p. 36.

38. Stapleton, pp. 34–35.

39. *AHBD*, p. 76.

40. Marie B. Allen Oral History Interview with Rachel Clark, Nov. 9, 1978.

41. *AHBD*, pp. 33–34.

42. David Alsobrook Oral History Interview with Lillian Carter, Sept. 26, 1978.

43. Ibid.

44. *AHBD*, p. 34.

45. Ibid., pp. 186–187.

46. Ibid., pp. 56–57.

47. Ibid., pp. 187–188

48. David Alsobrook Oral History Interview with Lillian Carter, Sept. 26, 1978.

49. *ML&F*, pp. 21–22.

50. David Alsobrook Oral History Interview with Lillian Carter, Sept. 26, 1978.

51. Coombs, p. 42.

52. William Carter, *Billy Carter: A Journey Through the Shadows* (Atlanta: Longstreet, 1999), p. 98

53. Coombs, p. 42.

54. Dr. Martin Luther King, Jr., Illinois Wesleyan Convocation, Feb. 10, 1966.

55. *AHBD*, p. 110.

56. Jimmy Carter, *Why Not the Best?* (New York: Bantam, 1976), p.41. Hereafter *WNTB?*

57. David Alsobrook Oral History Interview with Lillian Carter, Sept. 26, 1978.

58. Ibid.

59. *ML&F*, p. 16.

60. Ibid.

61. David Alsobrook Oral History Interview with Lillian Carter, Sept. 26, 1978.

62. *ARM*, p. 31.

63. Ibid., pp. 30–31; Andrew J. Young to author, Oct. 11, 2012.

64. James R. Gaines and Joyce Leviton, "Divided They Stand: A Portrait of Plains Bares the Roots of 'Billygate,'" *People Magazine*, Aug. 17, 1980.

65. *AHBD*, p. 265.

66. Stanley Godbold, *Jimmy & Rosalynn Carter: The Georgia Years, 1924–1974* (Oxford: Oxford University Press, 2010), p. 54.

67. Stapleton, p. 50.

68. HABS No. GA-2207, pp. 2, 6.

69. Ibid., p. 2.

70. Stapleton, p. 56.

71. David Alsobrook Oral History Interview with Lillian Carter, Sept. 26, 1978.

72. Rosalynn Carter, *First Lady from Plains* (New York: Houghton Mifflin, 1984), p. 11 (hereafter *FLFP*); Pousner, *The Atlanta Journal-Constitution*, Mar. 8, 2011.

73. *FLFP*, p. 10.

74. Ibid, p. 14.

75. Ibid., p. 15.

76. Ibid., p. 16.

77. Ibid., p. 19.

78. Huh Carter, *Cousin Beedie and Cousin Hot: My Life with the Carter Family of Plains, Georgia* (New York: Prentice-Hall, 1978), p. 63.

79. *FLFP*, p. 19.

80. Rick Hutto interview with author, June 18, 2011.

81. *ML&F*, p. 28.

Chapter 4

1. David Alsobrook Oral History Interview with Lillian Carter, Sept. 26, 1978.

2. *ML&F*, p. 34.

3. David Alsobrook Oral History Interview with Lillian Carter, Sept. 26, 1978.

4. Ibid.

5. Stapleton, p. 51.

6. Ibid., pp. 53–54.

7. David Alsobrook Oral History Interview with Lillian Carter, Sept. 26, 1978.

8. Stapleton, p. 54.

9. *ARM*, p. 74.

10. Stapleton, p. 54.

11. David Alsobrook Oral History Interview with Lillian Carter, Sept. 26, 1978.

12. *AHBD*, p. 258.

13. Stapleton, p. 55.

14. Ibid.

15. *AHBD*, p. 74.

16. Kim Carter Fuller to author, Mar. 11, 2011.

17. Stapleton, p. 55.

18. William Carter, p. 47.

19. Stapleton, p. 59.

20. Ibid., p. 56.

21. *ARM*, p. 78.

22. Ibid.

23. *ML&F*, p. 7

24. Jimmy Carter in conversation with author, Mar. 11, 2011.

25. *ARM*, p. 79.

26. "Lillian Carter Talks About Racism,

the Kennedys, and 'Jimmy's Reign,'" *Ms. Magazine*, October 1976.

27. Stapleton, p. 6.

28. Lillian Carter application to Kappa Alpha, collection of Kim Carter Fuller.

29. Tom Burson to author, Apr. 3, 2011.

30. Jim Rogers to author, Apr. 16, 2011.

31. *ML&F*, p. 8.

32. Sam Ligon to author, Apr. 10, 2011.

33. http://www.kappaalphaorder.org/.

34. Anthony James, "Political Parties: College Social Fraternities, Manhood, and the Defense of Southern Traditionalism, 1945–1960," in *White Masculinity in the Recent South*, edited by Trent Watts (Baton Rouge: Louisiana State University Press, 2008), pp. 70–75. The Kappa Alpha flag was finally retired in 1992. See John M. Coski, *The Confederate Battle Flag: America's Most Embattled Emblem* (Cambridge: Harvard University, 2005), pp. 222–223.

35. Jerrold Packard, *American Nightmare: The History of Jim Crow* (New York: Macmillan, 2003), p. 232.

36. Tom Burson to author, Apr. 3, 2011.

37. Tommy Morgan to author, Apr. 3, 2011.

38. Sam Ligon to author, Mar. 10, 2011.

39. Earl Wilson, *Milwaukee Sentinel*, Jan. 15, 1977, p. 22.

40. Jim Rogers to author, Apr. 16, 2011.

41. Tommy Morgan to author, Apr. 3, 2011.

42. Ibid.

43. *ML&F*, p. 8.

44. Tommy Morgan to author, Apr. 3, 2011.

45. Jim Rogers to author, Apr. 16, 2011.

46. Richard Hyatt *The Carters of Plains* (Huntsville: The Strode Publishers, 1977), p. 205.

47. Tommy Morgan to author, Apr. 3, 2011.

48. Jim Rogers to author, Apr. 16, 2011.

49. Ibid.

50. Bill Jordan to author, Apr. 8, 2011.

51. *ML&F*, p. 8.

52. Tommy Morgan to author, Apr. 3, 2011.

53. Sam Ligon to author, Apr. 10, 2011.

54. Tommy Morgan to author, Apr. 3, 2011.

55. Tom Burson to author, Apr. 3, 2011.

56. Tommy Morgan to author, Apr. 3, 2011.

57. Bill Jordan to author, Apr. 8, 2011.

58. Tommy Morgan to author, Apr. 3, 2011.

59. Ibid.

60. Sam Ligon to author, Apr. 10, 2011.

61. "Lillian Carter Talks About Racism, the Kennedys, and 'Jimmy's Reign,'" *Ms. Magazine*, October 1976, p. 51; Laura Holloway, "'Miss Lilly' Left for Some Sleep," *The Opelika-Auburn News*, Oct. 24, 1976.

62. Jimmy Carter, *The Virtues of Aging* (New York: Ballantine, 1998), p. 110.

63. Pousner, *The Atlanta Journal-Constitution*, Mar. 8, 2011.

64. Bill Jordan to author, Apr. 8, 2011.

65. *ML&F*, p. 9.

Chapter 5

1. Coombs, p. 43.

2. Robert Scheer, *Playing President: My Close Encounters with Nixon, Carter, Bush I, Reagan and Clinton—and How They Did Not Prepare Me for George W. Bush* (Brooklyn: Akashic Books, 2006), pp. 114–115.

3. Coombs, p. 43.

4. Clennon L. King to author, June 30, 2011.

5. Lenny Jordan to author, July 5, 2011.

6. Coombs, p. 43.

7. Mazlish, p. 51.

8. Ibid., p. 52.

9. Ibid., p. 48; Robert MacNeil, "A Conversation with Miss Lillian," WNET, Oct. 12, 1977.

10. *ARM*, p. 80.

11. *AFH*, p. 65.

12. *ARM*, p. 83; *AFH*, p. 27.

13. *Ms. Mag*, p. 86

14. *ARM*, p. 81

15. "Lillian Carter Talks About Racism, the Kennedys, and 'Jimmy's Reign,'" *Ms. Magazine*, October 1976, p. 86.

16. *ARM*, p. 81.

17. "Lillian Carter Talks About Racism, the Kennedys, and 'Jimmy's Reign,'" *Ms. Magazine*, October 1976, p. 86.

18. *ARM*, p. 82.

19. Ibid., p. 85.

20. Ibid.

21. Ibid.; Jimmy Carter, *Christmas in Plains: Memories* (New York: Simon & Schuster, 2001), p. 36.

22. *Stars & Stripes Magazine*, Dec. 25, 1966, p. 5.

23. "Lillian Carter Talks About Racism, the Kennedys, and 'Jimmy's Reign,'" *Ms. Magazine*, October 1976, p. 51; *ARM*, p. 83.

24. *ARM*, p. 83.

25. Kim Carter Fuller to author, Mar. 11, 2011.

26. *ARM*, p. 84.

27. Ibid., p. 85.

28. Kim Carter Fuller to author, Mar. 11, 2011.

29. *AFH*, p. 124.

30. Kim Carter Fuller to author, Mar. 11, 2011.

31. "Lillian Carter Talks About Racism, the Kennedys, and 'Jimmy's Reign,'" *Ms. Magazine*, October 1976, p. 51.

32. *AFH*, p. 153.

33. "Lillian Carter Talks About Racism, the Kennedys, and 'Jimmy's Reign,'" *Ms. Magazine*, October 1976, p. 51.

34. *Stars & Stripes Magazine*, Dec. 25, 1966, p. 5; Mike Douglas, WCHA # C-14, 13 December 1976/1000, CBS, "Mike Douglas Show with Lillian and Amy Carter in Plains: A Tour Through Plains," Jimmy Carter Library.

35. http://www.peacecorps.gov/index.cfm?shell=about.history.speech.

36. *ARM*, p. 87.

37. "Lillian Carter Talks About Racism, the Kennedys, and 'Jimmy's Reign,'" *Ms. Magazine*, October 1976, p. 52.

38. Ibid.

39. *AFH*, p. 10.

40. Larry Brown to author, Oct. 25, 2011.

41. Carol Stahl to author, Oct. 25, 2011.

42. Gabriel and Ruth Ross to author, Oct. 25, 2011.

43. *AFH*, p. 11.

44. "Lillian Carter Talks About Racism, the Kennedys, and 'Jimmy's Reign,'" *Ms. Magazine*, October 1976, p. 52.

45. Larry Brown to author, Oct. 25, 2011; *AFH*, p. 12.

46. Carmen Kagal, "Lillian Carter Revisits Vikhroli," *SPAN Magazine*, 1977. Hereafter Kagal.

47. *AFH*, pp. 11–12.

48. Van Shuler letter, Sept. 17, 1966.

49. *AFH*, p. 19.

50. Larry Brown to author, Oct. 15, 2011.

51. *AFH*, p. 53.

52. Larry Brown to author, Oct. 15, 2011.

53. Carol Stahl to author, Oct. 23, 2011.

54. Van Shuler to author, Nov. 19, 2011.

55. Larry Brown to author, Oct. 15, 2011; *AFH*, p. 21.

56. Carol Stahl et al., *We Asked Ourselves* (Bozeman: Carol Stahl, 2011), p. 15. Hereafter *WAO*.

57. *AFH*, p. 25.

58. Van Shuler letter, Oct. 7, 1966.

59. Jules Quinlan to author, Nov. 26, 2011.

60. *AFH*, p. 20, 25.

61. Ibid., p. 27.

62. Gabriel and Ruth Ross to author, Oct. 22, 2011.

63. Ibid.

64. *AFH*, p. 21.

65. Gabriel and Ruth Ross to author, Oct. 22, 2011.

66. Carol Stahl to author, Oct. 23, 2011.

67. Gabriel and Ruth Ross to author, Oct. 22, 2011; *AFH*, p. 28.

68. *AFH*, pp. 22–23.

69. Carol Stahl to author, Oct. 23, 2011.

70. *WAO*, p. 16.

71. Larry Brown to author, Oct. 16, 2011.

72. *AFH*, p. 27.

73. Gabriel and Ruth Ross to author, Oct. 22, 2011.

74. *AFH*, pp. 22, 24–25.

75. "Lillian Carter Talks About Racism, the Kennedys, and 'Jimmy's Reign,'" *Ms. Magazine*, October 1976, p. 52.

76. *AFH*, p. 31.

77. Ibid., p. 35.

Chapter 6

1. "Mrs. Carter Introduced to India Snake Charmers," *The Tampa Times*, Dec. 12, 1966; *WAO*, p. 37.

2. *AFH*, pp. 36–37.

3. "Granny No Rocker, Joins Peace Corps," *San Antonio Express,* Sept. 6, 1966; *AFH*, p. 37.

4. *WAO*, p. 47.

5. S.N. Agarwala, "Family Planning Programs in India: Past Performance and Likely Future Growth." *Asian Survey* 7, No. 12 (Dec. 1967): 851–859.

6. Ved Mehta, *Portrait of India* (New Haven: Yale University Press, 1993), pp. 14–15.

7. Kathleen Frank, *Indira: The Life of Indira Nehru Gandhi* (New York: HarperCollins, 2002), p. 295.

8. *AFH*, pp. 41–42, 45.

9. Carol Stahl to author, Oct. 23, 2011.

10. Kagal.

11. "Lillian Carter Talks About Racism, the Kennedys, and 'Jimmy's Reign,'" *Ms. Magazine*, October 1976, p. 52.

12. *AFH*, p. 66; Carol Stahl to author, Oct. 23, 2011.

13. *AFH*, p. 103.

14. Ibid., p. 52.
15. Ibid., p. 81.
16. Ibid.; Clayborne Carson, *The Autobiography of Martin Luther King, Jr.* (New York: Grand Central, 1998), p. 131.
17. Ibid., pp. 105, 48, 57.
18. Kagal.
19. *AFH*, pp. 62, 57; Carol Stahl to author, Oct. 23, 2011.
20. *ARM*, pp. 99–100; Lillian Carter letter from Vikhroli, Apr. 22, 1967, Kim Carter Fuller Collection.
21. *AFH*, p. 61.
22. Ibid., p. 110.
23. Ibid., p. 62.
24. Ibid., p. 100.
25. Ibid., p. 110.
26. Kagal.
27. *AFH*, pp. 63, 85–86, 92.
28. Ibid., p. 77.
29. Ibid., pp. 76, 84, 88.
30. Ibid., p. 95.
31. "Lillian Carter Talks About Racism, the Kennedys, and 'Jimmy's Reign,'" *Ms. Magazine*, October 1976, p. 52.
32. V.S. Naipaul, *India: A Wounded Civilization* (New York: Alfred A. Knopf, 1977), p. 17.
33. "Lillian Carter Talks About Racism, the Kennedys, and 'Jimmy's Reign,'" *Ms. Magazine*, October 1976, pp. 52–53.
34. *AFH*, pp. 72–73, 76.
35. Ibid., p. 74.
36. Ibid., p. 83; Kagal.
37. Carter, *Always a Reckoning*, p. 21
38. Kagal.
39. *AFH*, pp. 75, 98; Lillian Carter letter to Mr. and Mrs. Billy Carter, Kim Carter Fuller Collection. The franked date is smudged but appears to read Jan. 29, 1967. This was a Sunday. Given that post offices could be open for business on Sundays, it would make sense that the "Saturday night" with which she heads the letter was the day before she mailed it.
40. Ibid., pp. 65, 71.
41. "Lillian Carter Talks About Racism, the Kennedys, and 'Jimmy's Reign,'" *Ms. Magazine*, October 1976, p. 52.
42. Ibid., pp. 52, 54; Carol Stahl email to author, Oct. 24, 2011.
43. Suketu Mehta, *Maximum City: Bombay Lost and Found* (New York: Vintage, 2005), p. 125.
44. *AFH*, pp. 61, 67.
45. Carol Stahl to author, Oct. 23, 2011;

Scott Yewell to author, Dec. 21, 2011; "'Miss Lillian' Visits Old Roommate Here" (undated); letter from Lillian Carter to Anne Yewell Ashton, May 19, 1978; Lillian Carter to employees at Carter Warehouse, Feb. 12, 1967, Kim Carter Fuller Collection. The account of Lillian Pickett derives from conversations with Kim Carter Fuller.
46. "Lillian Carter Talks About Racism, the Kennedys, and 'Jimmy's Reign,'" *Ms. Magazine*, October 1976, p. 53.
47. Ibid.; *AFH*, pp. 121–122, 134.
48. *AFH*, p. 83.
49. *ARM*, pp. 114–115.
50. Ibid.
51. "Lillian Carter Talks About Racism, the Kennedys, and 'Jimmy's Reign,'" *Ms. Magazine*, October 1976, p. 54
52. *ARM*, p. 116.
53. "Lillian Carter Talks About Racism, the Kennedys, and 'Jimmy's Reign,'" *Ms. Magazine*, October 1976, p. 54.
54. Ibid.
55. Ibid.
56. Kagal.
57. *AFH*, p. 121.
58. Ibid., p. 113.
59. Ibid., pp. 94, 96, 110.

Chapter 7

1. *AFH*, p. 119.
2. Ibid., p. 118.
3. Ibid., pp. 119–120.
4. Ibid., p. 120.
5. Ibid., p. 122.
6. Gabriel and Ruth Ross to author, Oct. 22, 2011.
7. *AFH*, p. 58.
8. Gabriel and Ruth Ross to author, Oct. 22, 2011.
9. Gibran, p. 9.
10. *AFH*, p. 106.
11. Ibid.
12. Ibid., p. 107.
13. Mahabharata: http://www.mahabharata online.com/translation/mahabharata_12a 143.php.
14. AFH, pp. 101–102; "Lady Rama Rau Dies," *New York Times*, July 20, 1987.
15. *AFH*, pp. 104–105.
16. Ibid, pp. 108–109.
17. Ibid., pp. 107–108.
18. Ibid., p. 112.
19. Ibid., p. 115.
20. Ibid., pp. 124, 130–131.

21. Ibid., p. 130.
22. *ARM*, pp. 109–110.
23. *AFH*, p. 142.
24. *ARM*, p. 111.
25. *AFM*, pp. 150–151, 155.
26. Ibid., pp. 134, 153.
27. Ibid., p. 154.
28. Kagal, SPAN Magazine, 1977
29. Gabriel and Ruth Ross to author, Oct. 22, 2011.
30. *ARM*, pp. 122–123.
31. *AFH*, p. 155.
32. Ibid., p. 84.
33. Kim Carter Fuller to author, Feb. 6, 2012.
34. *AFH*, p. 154.
35. Ibid., p. 15.
36. *FLFP*, p. 63.
37. "President Carter's Sister Just Plains Folks," *San Mateo Times*, Aug. 30, 1977.
38. "Lillian Carter Talks About Racism, the Kennedys, and 'Jimmy's Reign,'" *Ms. Magazine*, October 1976, p. 86.
39. *ARM*, p. 125
40. *AFH*, p.120
41. Ibid., p. 153

Chapter 8

1. *Parade Magazine*, June 5, 1977
2. *ARM*, pp. 126–127.
3. Judy Klemesrud, "I'm More Political Than Jimmy," *The Miami News*, Apr. 30, 1979, p. 60.
4. *FLFP*, p. 65.
5. Jan Williams to author, Mar. 10, 2011.
6. John Walker to author, Oct. 6, 2011.
7. Ibid.
8. *ARM*, p. 147.
9. *WNTB?*, p. 117.
10. David Alsobrook Oral History Interview with Emily Gordy Dolvin, June 28, 1979; *FLFP*, p. 77.
11. David Alsobrook Oral History Interview with Emily Gordy Dolvin, June 28, 1979.
12. Godbold, pp. 183–184.
13. Kim Carter Fuller to author, Mar. 11, 2011.
14. Hyatt, pp. 200–201.
15. *Playground Daily News*, Apr. 22, 1976.
16. Rick Hutto interview with author, June 18, 2011.
17. *ARM*, p. 64.
18. Jan Williams to author, Mar. 10, 2011.

19. http://www.livingroomcandidate.org/commercials/1976/bio.
20. Phyllis Battelle, "'Miss Lillian' Carter is not worried," *Anderson Daily Bulletin*, Apr. 19, 1976.
21. Jan Williams to author, Mar. 10, 2011; Larry Brown to author, Oct. 16, 2011; "Rose Kennedy without the hair dye," *Redbook Magazine*, Oct. 1976, p. 84.
22. Lenore Nicklin, "Where Jimmy Carter Is King," *Sydney Morning Herald*, June 24, 1976, p. 4.
23. Scheer, p. 110
24. Georgie Ann Geyer, *Los Angeles Times*, June 14, 1976.
25. *ARM*, pp. 146–147.
26. Carlene Cimons, "Miss Lillian Tackles the Big Apple," *Los Angeles Times*, July 14, 1976.
27. Walt Smith, "Jimmy Carter's Mother Is Proud of Him," *Sarasota Herald-Tribune*, Apr. 25, 1976.
28. Coombs, p. 40; Andrew J. Young to author, Oct. 11, 2012.
29. Ibid.
30. Ibid., pp. 42–43.
31. Scheer, p. 114.
32. Coombs, p. 43.

Chapter 9

1. Clemence, Nov. 9, 1976, p. 9; William Carter, *Billy Carter*, p. 131.
2. Hyatt, pp. 129–132.
3. *ARM*, pp. 150–151.
4. Richard Hyatt to author, Apr. 29, 2012.
5. *FLFP*, p. 146.
6. *ML&F*, pp. 207–211.
7. Hyatt, p. 134.
8. Richard Harden to author, Apr. 14, 2012.
9. William Carter, *Billy Carter*, p. 53; Billy Carter and Sybil Carter with Ken Estes, *Billy: Billy Carter's Reflections on His Struggle with Fame, Alcoholism and Cancer* (Newport, RI: Edgehill Publications, 1990), p. 77.
10. Rick Hutto to author, June 18, 2011; *Parade Magazine*, Oct. 16, 1977; William Carter, *Billy Carter*, pp. 131–132; Andrew J. Young to author, Oct. 11, 2012. Billy bought the station with a partner, P.J. Wise, whose wife became alarmed when Billy applied for a liquor license. Phil Wise, P.J.'s son, told his father that as a church deacon, and seeing how upset his mother was, it would be best if he pulled out of the deal. Billy convinced P.J. to

close with him, and he would buy him out shortly after. "So for a few days of its existence," laughs Phil Wise, "the gas station was beer-free." Phil Wise to author, Oct. 9, 2012.

11. William Carter, *Billy Carter*, pp. 131–132.

12. *ML&F*, pp. 217–223.

13. Steven Borns to author, Apr. 21, 2012.

14. *ML&F*, pp. 222–224. Award-winning photographer Diana Mara Henry shot some of the first images of Lillian just as the returns came in. Some of these can be seen at this University of Massachusetts web page: http://www.library.umass.edu/spcoll/exhibits/henry/domestic.html.

15. William Carter, *Billy Carter*, p. 161.

Chapter 10

1. *ARM*, pp. 157–158, 162.

2. Kim Carter Fuller to author, Mar. 11, 2011.

3. "Hugh Carter Draws Lillian's Ire," *Los Angeles Times*, May 8, 1978, p. A2; *ARM*, p. 162; Carter and Carter with Estes, *Billy*, p. 71.

4. *ARM*, pp. 167–168.

5. Ibid.

6. Rick Hutto to author, June 18, 2011. Jimmy Carter wrote me that "we kept alcoholic drinks in the White House for our family use, like gin and tonic on the Truman balcony, but we did not serve it at public social events."

7. Rex Granum to author, Apr. 24, 2012

8. *ARM*, p. 155.

9. Rex Granum to author, Apr. 24, 2012; Rick Hutto to author, June 18, 2011.

10. Rick Hutto to author, June 18, 2011.

11. *ARM*, pp. 168–169.

12. Rex Granum to author, Apr. 21, 2012.

13. *ARM*, pp. 168–169. Air Force Two had once been Air Force One; it was the plane on which Lyndon B. Johnson was sworn in as President as President Kennedy's body was taken back to Washington, D.C.

14. Rex Granum to author, Apr. 21, 2012.

15. *ARM*, pp. 168–169; "Lillian Carter Meets with India's Indira Gandhi," *Spartanburg Herald-Journal*, Feb. 14, 1977, p. A7; "'Miss Lillian' Changes Her Opinion of Gandhi," *The Victoria Advocate*, Feb. 16, 1977, p. 7A.

16. Rex Granum to author, Apr. 21, 2012.

17. *ARM*, pp. 168–169.

18. Ibid.

19. Kagal, *SPAN Magazine*, 1977.

20. Ibid.

21. Ibid.; *ARM*, pp. 169–170.

22. "Miss Lillian Visits Peace Corps Veteran," *Sarasota Journal*, July 21, 1977; "Mabel Yewell Joins the Peace Corps at 71; Finds a Lady from Georgia Is Her Roommate," *The Aegis*, Mar. 31, 1977; letter from Lillian Carter to Anne Yewell Ashton, May 19, 1978

23. Larry Brown to author, Oct. 16, 2011.

24. Ibid.

25. Gabriel and Ruth Ross to author, Oct. 22, 2011.

26. Ibid.

27. Ibid.

28. Ibid.

29. Ibid.

30. Ibid.

31. Ibid.

32. Ibid.

33. Statement by Mrs. Lillian Carter at the annual benefit gala dinner of the Greater Chicago Area Chapter of UNICEF, Wednesday, March 29, 1978; Carter, Lillian: Personal Appearances 1/78–9/78, Jimmy Carter Library.

34. Memorandum for Christine Dodson from Rick Hutto, July 22, 1977; Correspondence—Carter, Lillian 1977; Jimmy Carter Library.

35. *Plains Georgia Monitor*, June 11, 1978, p. 5; Carter, Lillian: Personal Appearances 1/78–9/78, Jimmy Carter Library; Speech by H.E. Sir Dawda Kairaba Jawara at Juffure on the Occasion of Visit of Miss Lillian Carter to the Gambia, 24–26 July 1978, p. 2; Gambia, Banjul 2/77–7/78, Jimmy Carter Library.

36. Rick Hutto to author, June 18, 2011; "Miss Lillian to Take Hunger Tour," *The Milwaukee Sentinel*, July 13, 1978, p. 2.

37. "Miz Lillian Will Visit Drought Area," *The Hour*, July 20, 1978, p. 7.

38. "Miss Lillian feels for sand in her shoes," *The Afro-American*, July 29, 1978, p. 2.

39. Interview with Arthur M. Fell, Feb. 15, 1997, http://memory.loc.gov/service/mss/mssmisc/mfdip/2005%20txt%20files/2004fel03.txt.

40. "Miz Lillian Will Visit Drought Area," *The Hour*, Jul 20, 1978, p. 7; *Santa Ana Register*, Jul 27, 1978, p. A5

41. "Lillian Carter Given Medal," *Sarasota Herald-Tribune*, July 22, 1978, p. 11; Draft Statement for Miss Lillian's Remarks to the Food and Agriculture Organization;

FL 5–6 First Lady/Family-Lillian Carter, 5/1/78–1/20/81; Jimmy Carter Library.

42. Lillian also had dinner at Castel Sant' Angelo, originally the mausoleum of Emperor Hadrian, with Tina Anselmi, Minister of Health and first female cabinet minister, who like President Pertini had been a member of the resistance. "Lillian Carter gets honor medal," *The New Mexican*, July 21, 1978, p. A5.

43. Gardner, pp. 191–192.

44. Ibid.; "Lillian Carter Reflects on Audience with Pope," *Altoona Mirror*, July 24, 1978.

45. "Lillian Carter Meets Pope Paul," *St. Petersburg Times*, July 24, 1978, p. 5.

46. *The Georgia Bulletin*, Sept. 7, 1978.

47. *ARM*, pp. 180, 182–183.

48. "President's Mother Talks About Her Favorite Stars," *Jet*, Feb. 10, 1977, p. 52; Joy Billington, "This trip was no Peace Corps jaunt: Miz Lillian's slide show recalls the experience," *The Washington Star*, 1978.

49. "The President's Mother Goes to Africa," *Ebony*, October 1978, pp.164–170; Peace Corps *Action Update*, Sept. 21, 1978; letter from Lillian Carter to Mme. Caroline Diop, Dakar, August 1978; Senegal—Dakar [& Preceding Visit to Morocco by Lillian Carter] 2/77–8/78, Jimmy Carter Library.

50. Moneta Sleet, Jr., et al., "Miss Lillian in Africa: 'It Was So Emotional,'" *Jet*, Aug. 31, 1978, p. 12.

51. "Miss Lillian Visits Senegal," *Eugene Register-Guard*, July 26, 1978, p. 2.

52. Moneta Sleet, Jr., et al., "Miss Lillian in Africa: 'It Was So Emotional,'" *Jet*, Aug. 31, 1978, pp. 12–15

53. Ibid.

54. Carter, *Power Lines*, p. 277.

Chapter 11

1. Rex Granum to author, Apr. 21, 2012.

2. White House Communications Agency C514 Miss Lillian Composite, 14–21 November 1978, Jimmy Carter Library. A year before these talk show appearances, Lillian had a cameo role on a CBS Lucille Ball special, "Lucy Calls the President," which aired on November 21, 1977. Ball, who is frantically trying to prepare for a visit from President Carter but ends up destroying half her house and losing a front tooth, takes a call from Lillian, and the ensuing conversation is made nearly unintelligible by Ball's toothless speech impediment. As Ball struggles to communicate, Lillian gets in a zinger that would have made many a Southerner smile: "And they say *we* talk funny."

3. *The Hutchison News*, Nov. 11, 1977, p. 1.

4. "Miss Lillian Vows Hush on Policies," *The Anniston Star*, Feb. 19, 1980, p. 3A; *ARM*, pp. 187–189 and pp. 190–191.

5. Lillian Carter: Personal Appointments 1/78–9/78: Memorandum for Chairman John White from Tim Kraft and Richard Harden re: Campaign Appearances by Miss Lillian, 9–13–1978; Schedule of Trips for Miss Lillian, Saturday, September 16-Tuesday, September 19: Birmingham, AL, Little Rock, AR, and Emporia and Wichita, KS; Schedule of Trips for Miss Lillian, Sunday, September 24-Wednesday, September 17: Trenton, NJ, Long Island, NY, Westchester County, NY; The White House, Remarks of the President at Democratic National Committee Fundraiser, Page 1, Washington Hilton Hotel, 9–27–1978; *Argus-Leader*, Sept. 14, 1978.

6. Enid Nemy, *New York Times*, Dec. 2, 1977.

7. Andy Warhol, *The Andy Warhol Diaries*, ed. Pat Hackett (New York: Grand Central, 1991), pp. 73–74.

8. Paul Lewis, "Nani Palkhivala, 82, Dies; Civil Rights Leader in India," *New York Times*, Dec. 13, 2002.

9. Nemy, *New York Times*, Dec. 2, 1977.

10. "Miss Lillian steps out, "*Lawrence Journal-World*, Dec. 6, 1977, p. 4.

11. *Sarasota Herald-Tribune*, Dec. 13, 1977.

12. Steve Rubell interview with *INTERVIEW*, http://d30030908.purehost.com/id156.htm

13. "The Adventures of Miss Lillian," *The Victoria Advocate*, Oct. 5, 1978, p. 21.

14. Doug Shuit, "Lillian Carter At Gays' Dinner; $120,000 Raised," *Los Angeles Times*, Oct. 26, 1979, p. B3.

15. "Tom Cruise Outguns the Cowboy," *New York Daily News*, April 7, 2008, http://www.nydailynews.com/entertainment/gossip/tom-cruise-outguns-cowboy-article-1.279989.

16. Peter Shapiro, *Turn the Beat Around: The Secret History of Disco* (London: Faber and Faber, 2005), p. 181.

17. "Miss Lillian goes home," *The Tuscaloosa News*, May 1, 1977, p. 7.

18. *ARM*, p. 186.

19. Jan Williams to author, Mar. 11, 2011.

20. Ibid.

21. Ibid.

22. "Miss Lillian Is Back in Circulation," *Rome News-Tribune*, Jan. 16, 1977, p. 4.

23. *ARM*, p. 186.

24. "Miss Lillian goes home," *The Tuscaloosa News*, May 1, 1977, p. 7.

25. Jan Williams to author, Mar. 11, 2011.

26. Richard Hyatt to author, Apr. 29, 2012.

27. John Walker to author, Oct. 6, 2011.

28. Richard Hyatt to author, Apr. 29, 2012.

29. John Walker to author, Oct. 6, 2011.

30. Ibid.

31. Richard Hyatt to author, Apr. 29, 2012.

32. *Saturday Night Live* transcript for show aired Mar. 12, 1977, http://snltranscripts.jt.org/76/76o.phtml

33. John Walker to author, Oct. 6, 2011.

34. Ibid.

35. "Lillian here: I hate it in Miami," *The Miami News*, Aug. 29, 1979, p. 59.

36. "Miss Lillian Has Broken Hip," *Fort Scott Tribune*, Sept. 29, 1980, p. 36.

37. Jimmy Carter Diary entry for Oct. 3, 1980, http://www.jimmycarterlibrary.gov/documents/diary/1980/d100380t.pdf

38. "Miss Lillian Packs a Punch," *Indiana Evening Gazette*, Sept. 13, 1978.

39. Steven Hunsicker to author, Feb. 20, 2012

40. *ARM*, pp. 192–193.

41. "President's mother says Ayatollah should be killed," *Lawrence Journal-World*, Jan 30, 1979, p. 28; Justine De Lacey, "Miz Lillian: Hi, I'm Jimmy's Mother—A Candid Talk with the Carter Matriarch as She Paused in Paris," *International Herald Tribune*, April 19–20, 1980.

42. *ARM*, pp. 196–197.

43. "'Miss Lillian' Carter Dies of Cancer," *The Bryan Times*, Oct. 31, 1983, p. 1.

44. Kim Carter Fuller to author, Mar. 11, 2011.

45. "Sadat Visits Plains, GA; Carter Urges Fulfillment of Camp David Pledges," *Toledo Blade*, Aug. 10, 1981, p. 2.

46. "Carter and Begin Embrace in Plains, Ga," *Observer-Reporter*, Sept. 16, 1981, p. 7.

47. "Lillian Carter Undergoes Mastectomy," *Anchorage Daily News*, June 30, 1981, p. 4; David Bird and Alvin Krebs, "Lillian Carter Undergoes Mastectomy," *New York Times*, June 30, 1981.

48. "Ruth Carter Stapleton Dies of Cancer," *The Courier*, Sept. 27, 1983, p. 21.

49. *ARM*, pp. 204–205.

50. Ibid.

51. Kim Carter Fuller to author, Mar. 11, 2011; Carter and Carter with Estes, *Billy*, p. 72.

52. Ibid.

53. Rick Hutto to author, June 18, 2011.

54. Kim Carter Fuller to author, Mar. 11, 2011.

55. Ibid.

56. *Time Magazine*, Nov. 14, 1983

Epilogue

1. Kim Carter Fuller to author, Oct. 14, 2012.

2. Jimmy Carter, *Always a Reckoning and Other Poems*, p. 19.

Bibliography

Books

Agee, James, and Walker Evans. *Let Us Now Praise Famous Men*. New York: Mariner Books, 2001.

Anderson, Alan. *Remembering Americus: Essays on Southern Life*. Charleston: History Press, 2006.

Angelo, Bonnie. *First Mothers: The Women Who Shaped the Presidents*. New York: HarperCollins, 2001.

Arsenault, Raymond. *Freedom Riders: 1961 and the Struggle for Racial Justice*. Oxford: Oxford University Press, 2006.

Berlin, Ira. *Many Thousands Gone: The First Two Centuries of Slavery in North America*. New Haven: Harvard University Press, 1998.

Blackmon, Douglas. *Slavery by Another Name: The Re-Enslavement of Black Americans From the Civil War to World War II*. New York: Anchor Books, 2008.

Borns, Steven. *People of Plains, GA*. New York: McGraw-Hill, 1978.

Brinkley, Douglas. *The Unfinished Presidency: Jimmy Carter's Journey Beyond the White House*. New York: Penguin, 1998.

Brown, J. Larry. *Peasants Come Last: A Memoir of the Peace Corps at Fifty*. Sunnyvale: Lucita, 2011.

Carlton, David L., and Peter A. Coclanis. *Confronting Southern Poverty in the Great Depression: The Report on Economic Conditions of the South with Related Documents*. New York: Bedford/St. Martin's Press, 1996.

Carson, Clayborne, ed. *The Autobiography of Martin Luther King, Jr.* New York: Grand Central, 1998.

Carter, Billy, and Sybil Carter with Ken Estes. *Billy: Billy Carter's Reflections on His Struggle with Fame, Alcoholism and Cancer*. Newport, RI: Edgehill Publications, 1990.

Carter, Hugh. *Cousin Beedie and Cousin Hot: My Life with the Carter Family of Plains, Georgia*. New York: Prentice-Hall, 1978.

Carter, Jason. *Power Lines: Two Years on South Africa's Borders*. Washington, D.C.: National Geographic Society, 2002.

Carter, Jeff. *Ancestors of Jimmy and Rosalynn Carter*. Jefferson: McFarland, 2012.

Carter, Jimmy. *Always a Reckoning and Other Poems*. New York: Random House, 1995.

_____. *Beyond the White House: Waging Peace, Fighting Disease, Building Hope*. New York: Simon & Schuster, 2007.

_____. *Christmas in Plains: Memories*. New York: Simon & Schuster, 2001.

_____. *An Hour Before Daylight: Memories of a Rural Boyhood*. New York: Simon & Schuster, 2001.

_____. *Keeping Faith: Memoirs of a President*. New York: Bantam, 1982.

_____. *Living Faith*. New York: Crown, 1996.

_____. *Our Endangered Values: America's Moral Crisis*. New York: Simon & Schuster, 2005.

_____. *A Remarkable Mother*. New York: Simon & Schuster, 2008.

_____. *The Virtues of Aging*. New York: Ballantine, 1998.

_____. *Why Not the Best?* New York: Bantam, 1976.

Carter, Lillian, with Gloria Carter Spann. *Away From Home: Letters to My Family*. New York: Simon & Schuster, 1977.

Carter, Rosalynn. *First Lady from Plains*. New York: Houghton Mifflin, 1984.

Carter, William. *Billy Carter: A Journey Through the Shadows*. Atlanta: Longstreet, 1999.

Clinton, Catherine. *Tara Revisited: Women, War, & the Plantation Legend*. New York: Abbeville Press, 1995.

Coski, John M. *The Confederate Battle Flag: America's Most Embattled Emblem*. Cambridge: Harvard University, 2005.

Dubois, W.E. B. *The Souls of Black Folk*. New York: Barnes & Noble Classics, 2003.

Frank, Kathleen. *Indira: The Life of Indira Nehru Gandhi*. New York: HarperCollins, 2002.

Gandhi, Mohandas. *Gandhi On Non-Violence: Selected Texts from Mohandas K. Gandhi*. Ed. Thomas Merton. New York: New Directions, 1965.

George, Nelson. *Where Did Our Love Go? The Rise & Fall of the Motown Sound*. Sydney: Omnibus Press, 1987.

Godbold, Stanley. *Jimmy & Rosalynn Carter: The Georgia Years, 1924–1974*. Oxford: Oxford University Press, 2010.

Gullam, Harold I. *Faith of Our Mothers: The Stories of Presidential Mothers from Mary Washington to Barbara Bush*. Grand Rapids: William B. Eerdmans, 2001.

Halliburton, Richard. *The Royal Road to Romance*. Palo Alto: Travelers Tales Classics, Publishers Groups West, 2000.

Hyatt, Richard. *The Carters of Plains*. Huntsville: The Strode Publishers, 1977.

James, Anthony. "Political Parties: College Social Fraternities, Manhood, and the Defense of Southern Traditionalism, 1945–1960," in *White Masculinity in the Recent South*, ed. Trent Watts. Baton Rouge: Louisiana State University Press, 2008.

Jones, Henry Z. *More Palatine Families*. Marco Island, FL: Picton Press, 1991.

Lee, Dallas. *The Cotton Patch Evidence: The Story of Clarence Jordan and the Koinonia Farm Experiment*. New York: Harper & Row, 1971.

Mazlish, Bruce, and Edwin Diamond. *Jimmy Carter: A Character Portrait*. New York: Simon & Schuster, 1979.

Mehta, Suketu. *Maximum City: Bombay Lost and Found*. New York: Vintage, 2005.

Mehta, Ved. *Portrait of India*. New Haven: Yale University Press, 1993.

Meisler, Stanly. *When the World Calls: Inside the Peace Corps and Its First Fifty Years*. Boston: Beacon Press, 2011.

Mitchell, Stephen, transl. *Baghavad Gita: A New Translation*. New York: Harmony Books, 2000.

Mohanti, Prafulla. *My Village, My Life: Portrait of an Indian Village*. Westport, CT: Praeger, 1974.

Naipaul, V. S. *India: A Wounded Civilization*. New York: Alfred A. Knopf, 1977.

_____. *A Turn in the South*. New York: Vintage, 1989.

Neiman, LeRoy. *All Told: My Art and Life Among Athletes, Playboys, Bunnies, and Provocateurs*. Guilford, CT: Lyons Press, 2012.

Packard, Jerrold. *American Nightmare: The History of Jim Crow*. New York: Macmillan, 2003.

Roberts, Cokie. *Founding Mothers: The Women Who Raised Our Nation*. New York: William Morrow, 2004.

Roberts, Gary Boyd. *Ancestors of American Presidents*. Boston: New England Historic Genealogical Society, 2009.

Scheer, Robert. *Playing President: My Close Encounters with Nixon, Carter, Bush I, Reagan and Clinton—and How They Did Not Prepare Me for George W. Bush*. Brooklyn: Akashic Books, 2006.

Shapiro, Peter. *Turn the Beat Around: The Secret History of Disco*. London: Faber and Faber, 2005.

Stahl, Carol, et al. *We Asked Ourselves: An Anthology of Answers by India 39 Returned Peace Corps Volunteers*. Bozeman: Carol Stahl, 2011.

Stapleton, Ruth Carter. *Brother Billy*. New York: HarperCollins, 1978.

Strawser, Nina. "A Prescription for Peace." Nina Strawser Papers, 1967.

_____. "A Tribute to My Era." Nina Strawser Papers, 1970.

Chinmayananda. *The Art of Living*. Mumbai: Central Chinmaya Mission Trust, 2009.

Tartan, Beth, and Rudy Hayes. *Miss Lillian and Friends: The Plains, Georgia Family Philosophy and Recipe Book*. New York: Signet, 1977.

Tuck, Stephen G. N. *Beyond Atlanta: The Struggle for Racial Equality in Georgia, 1940–1980*. Athens: University of Georgia Press, 2003.

Warhol, Andy. *The Andy Warhol Diaries*. Ed. Pat Hackett. New York: Grand Central, 1991.

Watkins, T. H. *The Great Depression: America in the 1930s.* Boston: Back Bay Books, 2009.

Wead, Doug. *The Raising of a President: The Mothers and Fathers of Our Nation's Leaders.* New York: Atria, 2005.

Wiser, William H., and Charlotte Viall Wiser. *Behind Mud Walls: 1930–1960.* Berkeley: University of California Press, 1971.

Wooten, James. *Dasher: The Roots and Rising of Jimmy Carter.* New York: Simon & Schuster, 1978.

Oral Histories

Allen, Marie B. Oral History Interview with Fanny Surasky Gordy, Feb. 11, 1980, Jimmy Carter Library.

Allen, Marie B. Oral History Interview with Rachel Clark, Nov. 9, 1978, Jimmy Carter Library.

Alsobrook, David. Oral History Interview with Elizabeth Gordy Braunstein, Nov. 14, 1979, Jimmy Carter Library.

Alsobrook, David. Oral History Interview with Emily Gordy Dolvin, June 28, 1979, Jimmy Carter Library.

Alsobrook, David. Oral History Interview with Lillian Carter, Sept. 26, 1978, Jimmy Carter Library

Articles

"The Adventures of Miss Lillian." *The Victoria Advocate,* Oct. 5, 1978.

Agarwala, S.N. "Family Planning Programs in India: Past Performance and Likely Future Growth." *Asian Survey* 7, no. 12 (Dec. 1967).

Anderson, Jack. "Miss Lillian wins Italian President's favor." *Deseret News,* Aug. 2, 1978.

Baker, Shamim M., Otis W. Brawley, and Leonard S. Marks. "Effects of Untreated Syphilis in the Negro Male, 1932 to 1972: A Closure Comes to the Tuskegee Study, 2004." Urology 65(6), 2005.

Battelle, Phyllis. "'Miss Lillian' Carter is not worried." *Anderson Daily Bulletin,* Apr. 19, 1976.

Billington, Joy. "This trip was no Peace Corps jaunt: Miz Lillian's slide show recalls the experience." *The Washington Star,* 1978.

Bird, David, and Alvin Krebs. "Lillian Carter Undergoes Mastectomy." *New York Times,* June 30, 1981.

Brinkley, Douglas. "A Time for Reckoning: Jimmy Carter and the Cult of Kinfolk." *Presidential Studies Quarterly* (1999).

"Carter and Begin Embrace in Plains, Ga." *Observer-Reporter,* Sept. 16, 1981.

"Carter Gets His 'Good Points' from Her, Says Miss Lillian." *Sarasota Herald-Tribune,* July 22, 1978.

Carter, Lillian. *Guideposts,* December 1977.

Cimons, Carlene. "Miss Lillian Tackles the Big Apple." *Los Angeles Times,* July 14, 1976.

Coombs, Orde. "The Hand That Rocked Carter's Cradle." *New York Magazine,* June 14, 1976.

De Lacey, Justine. "Miz Lillian: Hi, I'm Jimmy's Mother—A Candid Talk with the Carter Matriarch as She Paused in Paris." *International Herald Tribune,* April 19–20, 1980.

Gaines, James R., and Joyce Leviton. "Divided They Stand: A Portrait of Plains Bares the Roots of 'Billygate.'" *People* Magazine, Aug. 17, 1980.

The Georgia Bulletin, Sept. 7, 1978.

Geyer, Georgie Ann. *Los Angeles Times,* June 14, 1976.

"Granny No Rocker, Joins Peace Corps." *San Antonio Express,* Sept. 6, 1966.

Holloway, Laura. "'Miss Lilly' Left for Some Sleep." *The Opelika-Auburn News,* Oct. 24, 1976.

"Hugh Carter Draws Lillian's Ire." *Los Angeles Times,* May 8, 1978.

The Hutchison News, Nov. 11, 1977.

Kagal, Carmen. "Lillian Carter Revisits Vikhroli." *SPAN,* 1977.

Klemesrud, Judy. "I'm More Political Than Jimmy." *The Miami News,* Apr. 30, 1979.

"Lady Rama Rau Dies." *New York Times,* July 20, 1987.

Lewis, Paul. "Nani Palkhivala, 82, Dies; Civil Rights Leader in India." *New York Times,* Dec 13, 2002.

"Lillian Carter gets honor medal." *The New Mexican,* July 21,1978.

"Lillian Carter Given Medal." *Sarasota Herald-Tribune,* July 22, 1978.

"Lillian Carter Meets Pope Paul." *St. Petersburg Times,* July 24, 1978.

"Lillian Carter Meets with India's Indira Gandhi." *Spartanburg Herald-Journal,* Feb. 14, 1977.

"Lillian Carter Reflects on Audience with Pope." *Altoona Mirror,* July 24, 1978.

"Lillian Carter Talks About Racism, the

Kennedys, and 'Jimmy's Reign.'" *Ms. Magazine*, October 1976.

"Lillian Carter Undergoes Mastectomy." *Anchorage Daily News*, June 30, 1981.

"Lillian here: I hate it in Miami." *The Miami News*, Aug. 29, 1979.

MacNeil, Robert. "A Conversation with Miss Lillian." *WNET*, Oct 12, 1977.

"Mabel Yewell Joins the Peace Corps at 71; Finds a Lady from Georgia Is Her Roommate." *The Aegis*, Mar. 31, 1977.

Michaels, Marguerite. "Will the Presidency Spoil the Carter Family?" *Parade Magazine*, Oct. 16, 1977.

"Miss Lillian and Miss Allie Talk Post Office." *Postal Life*, March/April 1977.

"'Miss Lillian' Carter Dies of Cancer." *The Bryan Times*, Oct. 31, 1983.

"'Miss Lillian' Changes Her Opinion of Gandhi." *The Victoria Advocate*, Feb. 16, 1977.

"Miss Lillian feels for sand in her shoes." *The Afro-American*, July 29, 1978.

"Miss Lillian goes home." *The Tuscaloosa News*, May 1, 1977.

"Miss Lillian Has Broken Hip." *Fort Scott Tribune*, Sep 29, 1980.

"Miss Lillian Is Back in Circulation." *Rome News-Tribune*, Jan. 16, 1977.

"Miss Lillian Packs a Punch." *Indiana Evening Gazette*, Sept. 13, 1978.

"Miss Lillian steps out." *Lawrence Journal-World*, Dec. 6, 1977.

"Miss Lillian to Take Hunger Tour." *The Milwaukee Sentinel*, July 13, 1978.

"Miss Lillian Visits Peace Corps Veteran." *Sarasota Journal*, July 21, 1977.

"Miss Lillian Visits Senegal." *Eugene Register-Guard*, July 26, 1978.

"Miss Lillian Vows Hush on Policies." *The Anniston Star*, Feb 19,1980.

"Mr. D.C. Gordy Ends His Life; Sad Death of a Prominent Citizen of Chattahoochee." *Columbus Daily Enquirer*, Nov. 13, 1902.

"Miz Lillian Will Visit Drought Area." *The Hour*, July 20, 1978.

"Mrs. Carter Introduced to India Snake Charmers." *The Tampa Times*, Dec. 12, 1966.

Nemy, Enid. *New York Times*, Dec. 2, 1977.

Nicklin, Lenore. "Where Jimmy Carter Is King." *Sydney Morning Herald*, Jun 24, 1976.

Parade Magazine, June 5, 1977.

Peace Corps *Action Update*, Sept. 21, 1978.

Plains Georgia Monitor, June 11, 1978.

Playground Daily News, Apr. 22, 1976.

Pousner, Howard. *The Atlanta Journal-Constitution*, Mar 8, 2011.

"President Carter, Wife, Honor 'Miss Lillian.'" *Macon News*, March 10, 2011.

"President Carter's Sister Just Plains Folks." *San Mateo Times*, Aug. 30, 1977.

"The President's Mother Goes to Africa." *Ebony*, October 1978.

"President's mother says Ayatollah should be killed." *Lawrence Journal-World*, Jan. 30, 1979.

"President's Mother Talks About Her Favorite Stars." *Jet*, Feb. 10, 1977.

Redbook Magazine, Oct. 1976.

"Ruth Carter Stapleton Dies of Cancer." *The Courier*, Sept. 27, 1983.

"Sadat Visits Plains, GA; Carter Urges Fulfillment of Camp David Pledges." *Toledo Blade*, Aug. 10, 1981.

Santa Ana Register, July 27, 1978.

Shuit, Doug. "Lillian Carter At Gays' Dinner; $120,000 Raised." *Los Angeles Times*, Oct. 26, 1979.

Sleet, Jr., Moneta, et al. "Miss Lillian in Africa: 'It Was So Emotional.'" *Jet*, Aug. 31, 1978.

Smith, Walt. "Jimmy Carter's Mother Is Proud of Him." *Sarasota Herald-Tribune*, Apr. 25, 1976.

"The Spirited Matriarch from Plains." *Time Magazine*, Nov. 14, 1983.

Stars & Stripes Magazine, Dec. 25, 1966.

Thomas, Jr., Kenneth H. *Georgia Life*, Winter 1976 and Spring 1980.

Wilson, Earl. *Milwaukee Sentinel*, Jan. 15, 1977.

Primary Sources

Carter, Lillian. Application to Kappa Alpha, Kim Carter Fuller Collection.

_____. Draft letter to Mme, Caroline Diop, Dakar, August 1978, Senegal—Dakar [& Preceding Visit to Morocco by Lillian Carter] Feb. 1977-Aug. 1978, Jimmy Carter Library.

_____. Draft statement for Miss Lillian's Remarks to the Food and Agriculture Organization, FL 5–6 First Lady/Family-Lillian Carter, May 1, 1978–Jan. 20, 1981, Jimmy Carter Library.

_____. Letter from Vikhroli, Apr. 22, 1967, Kim Carter Fuller Collection.

_____. Letter to employees at Carter Warehouse, Feb. 12, 1967: Kim Carter Fuller Collection.

_____. Letter to Mr. and Mrs. Billy Carter (Jan. 29, 1967?): Kim Carter Fuller Collection.

_____. Personal Appearances 1/78–9/78, Jimmy Carter Library.

_____. Statement by Mrs. Lillian Carter at the annual benefit gala dinner of the Greater Chicago Area Chapter of UNICEF, Wednesday, Mar. 29, 1978; Carter, Lillian: Personal Appearances Jan. 1978–Sept. 1978, Jimmy Carter Library.

Hutto, Rick. Memorandum for Christine Dodson from Rick Hutto, July 22, 1977; Correspondence—Carter, Lillian 1977; Jimmy Carter Library.

Jawara, Sir Dawda Kairaba. Speech by H.E. Sir Dawda Kairaba Jawara at Juffure on the Occasion of Visit of Miss Lillian Carter to the Gambia: 24–26 July 1978, Gambia, Banjul, Feb. 1977–July 1978, Jimmy Carter Library.

Shuler, Evangeline. Letters from India, Sept. 17, 1966, Oct. 7, 1966, Van Shuler Papers.

Watson, Tom. Letter to James Jackson Gordy, Jan. 6, 1916. University of North Carolina Library.

Video

Carter, Lillian. White House Communications Agency C514 Miss Lillian Composite (Merv Griffin and Dinah Shore), Nov. 14–21, 1978; Jimmy Carter Library.

The Mike Douglas Show. Mike Douglas, WCHA #C-14, Dec. 13, 1976/1000, CBS, "Mike Douglas Show with Lillian and Amy Carter in Plains: A Tour Through Plains," Jimmy Carter Library.

Web

The Arts & Crafts Society. "Sears, Roebuck Houses Offered between 1908 and 1940," http://www.arts-crafts.com/archive/sears-roebuck.shtml.

The Association for Diplomatic Studies and Training Foreign Affairs Oral History Project. Interview with Arthur M. Fell, W. Haven North, Feb, 15, 1997, http://memory.loc.gov/service/mss/mssmisc/mfdip/2005%20txt%20files/2004fel03.txt.

Jimmy Carter Diary entry, Oct. 3, 1980, http://www.jimmycarterlibrary.gov/documents/diary/1980/d100380t.pdf

Kappa Alpha Order, http://www.kappaalphaorder.org/.

King, Jr., Dr. Martin Luther. Illinois Wesleyan Convocation, Feb. 10,1966 https://www.iwu.edu/news/2006/KingSpeech1.html.

Mahabarata, Santi Parva, Section CXLIV, trans. Kisari Mohan Ganguli, http://www.mahabharataonline.com/translation/mahabharata_12a143.php.

Museum of the Moving Image. The Living Room Candidate, Presidential Campaign Commercials 1952–2012, Carter vs. Ford 1976, http://www.livingroomcandidate.org/commercials/1976/bio.

Peace Corps. Remarks of Senator John F. Kennedy, http://www.peacecorps.gov/index.cfm?shell=about.history.speech.

Saturday Night Live. Transcript for Mar. 12, 1977, http://snltranscripts.jt.org/76/76o.phtml.

"Tom Cruise Outguns the Cowboy." New York Daily News, April 7, 2008, http://www.nydailynews.com/entertainment/gossip/tom-cruise-outguns-cowboy-article-1.279989.

Interviews

Alsobrook, David. June 2011.

Bhatia, Dr. Gyansham. Jan. 2011.

Borns, Steven. Apr. 2012.

Brown, Larry. Oct. 2011.

Burson, Tom. Apr. 2011.

Carter, Jack and Elizabeth. June 2012.

Carter, Jimmy. 2011–2012.

Daschle, Sen. Tom. Dec. 2012.

Fuller, Kim Carter. Mar. 2011, June 2011, Feb. 2012, Oct. 2012.

Granum, Rex. Apr. 2012.

Harden, Richard. Apr. 2012.

Hunsicker, Steven. Feb. 2012

Hutto, Richard. June 2011.

Hyatt, Richard. Apr. 2012.

Jordan, Bill. Apr. 2011.

Jordan, Lenny. July 2011.

Ligon, Sam. Apr. 2011.

Morgan, Tommy. Apr. 2011.

Pethe, Madhavi. Apr. 2011, Oct. 2011, Jan. 2012.

Quinlan, Jules. Nov. 2011.

Rogers, Jim. Apr. 2011.

Ross, Gabriel and Ruth. Oct. 2011.

Shuler, Van. Nov. 2011.

Stahl, Carol. Oct. 2011.

Walker, John. Oct. 2011.

Williams, Jan. Mar. 2011.

Wise, Phil. Oct. 2012.

Yewell, Scott. Dec. 2011.

Young, Andrew J. Oct. 2012.

Index